ANATOMY OF A YES

FIELD NOTES FROM AN ORGAN DONATION ADVOCATE IN APPALACHIA

BRENT WHETSTONE

CONTENTS

DISCLAIMER

The stories and cases presented in this book are based on the author's professional experiences in the field of organ donation advocacy. In compliance with the Health Insurance Portability and Accountability Act (HIPAA) and other applicable privacy laws, all identifying information has been altered, and certain cases have been fictionalized or presented as composite scenarios to protect the privacy and confidentiality of the individuals involved. Any resemblance to specific persons, living or deceased, is purely coincidental.

The purpose of this work is to educate, inform, and advocate for greater understanding of organ donation, particularly within the Appalachian region, and not to disclose private or confidential health information.

DEDICATION

To Heather, my wife, my strength, my steadfast heart—
who faced breast cancer with grace and grit,
and who, even in her own battle, carried me through mine.
This book is as much her victory as it is mine.

To Caitlyn, Isabella, Noah, Madeline, and Abigail,
my beloved children—
who have shared me with the road, the hospital, and the grief of strangers.
Your patience, laughter, and love fill the silences between my work.

To the donor families,

who, in the midst of unspeakable loss, found the courage to say yes. You are the quiet heroes whose legacy this book seeks to honor.

To the reader,
Whether you are a healthcare professional, a family member, or simply someone seeking to understand the human side of donation—thank you. May these pages offer insight, invite compassion, and remind you that every "yes" comes from a sacred place of love, courage, and hope. You are part of that story now.

THE WHETSTONE FAMILY
FOUNDATION
ADVANCING MEDICINE AND THE ARTS

Anatomy of a Yes: Field Notes from an Organ Donation Advocate in Appalachia

Published by Inland Sea Press
Middlefield, Ohio, USA

ISBN 979-8218858353

For information, permissions, or bulk orders, contact:
Inland Sea Press
Email: info@inlandseapress.org

First Edition

Cover design and interior layout by Inland Sea Press
Printed in the United States of America

PROLOGUE
ONE MAN'S YES

I've been a trauma chaplain for just under ten years. Never in a million years did I imagine I'd spend my days in emergency departments and intensive care units.

The truth is, I hated hospitals. They unsettled me—the sights, the sounds, the smells. As a youth minister, I did everything I could to avoid hospital visitations. If I had to go, it usually meant walking into the worst kind of moment: a sick child, or worse, parents who had just been handed a devastating diagnosis—or the unthinkable news that their child had died.

But if I wanted to be successful in ministry—and if I truly wanted to provide the care my students and their families needed—I had to face my fear of hospitals and clinical settings. Everyone around me knew how much I dreaded those late-night calls.

One night, while I was talking with a friend about that very dread, the phone rang. I didn't even have to look at the caller ID; I knew what it was going to be. Another hospital call. Another crisis. My friend listened and then said something I hadn't considered before: *"You need to work through this. Have you ever heard of Clinical Pastoral Education[1]?"*

I had no idea what CPE was—or how being accepted into the program at Mercy Health would change the entire trajectory of my life. I couldn't have known that those long hours, hard conversations, and bedside prayers would lead me to my true calling: the sacred, often invisible work of being an Organ Donation Advocate.

At the time, I knew almost nothing about organ procurement. What little I *did* know came from medical dramas on television—which, I quickly discovered, is a terrible place to get your facts about this field.

It was during my first unit of CPE that we met the Hospital Development representative—the liaison between our hospital and the Organ Procurement Organization (OPO)[2]. She came to speak with our chaplain cohort, and that one conversation would plant a seed I didn't yet know was growing.

---

1 Clinical Pastoral Education (CPE) is a professional training program for spiritual care providers and chaplains that combines classroom learning with supervised clinical experience in hospitals or other healthcare settings. It emphasizes self-reflection, interfaith competency, and the development of skills to support individuals during crises, illness, grief, and trauma (Association for Clinical Pastoral Education, ACPE.edu).

2 An Organ Procurement Organization (OPO) is a federally designated nonprofit responsible for coordinating organ donation and transplantation within a specific geographic area. They work with hospitals, donor families, and transplant centers to recover and allocate organs for lifesaving transplants (U.S. Department of Health & Human Services, Health Resources & Services Administration. organdonor.gov).

In 2017, we were told that over 3,000 Ohioans were waiting for the life-saving gift of an organ. The Hospital Development coordinator broke it down for us:

2,400 were waiting on a kidney,

400 on a liver,

150 on a heart,

100 on lungs,

and around 50 on a pancreas or other organs.

"These are our friends, our relatives, our neighbors," she said. "All of them live right here in Ohio—waiting on someone to say yes."

At the time, I didn't think much of it. I went home and went about my evening like any other.

That night, as my wife and I often did, we sat down to watch an episode of *Grey's Anatomy*. The storyline centered on a child waiting for a transplant. *Grey's* always had a way of hitting you in the gut—this episode was no different.

I remember watching that scene and suddenly imagining myself in those parents' shoes.

What if it were one of our kids?

What if they were waiting—and no one said 'yes'?

That night, without fanfare or second-guessing, I logged on to www.donatelife.net and registered to be an organ, tissue, and eye donor.

A few months went by, and I was rounding on the neuro intensive care unit when I ran into the Hospital Development Coordinator again. She lit up when she saw me and said, "There's my chaplain friend!"

We exchanged a few pleasantries—she asked how I was doing with my studies and how the internship was going. Then, almost casually, she said, "Hey, want to see what brain death testing is like?"

I paused. I'd heard the doctors talk about brain death before—being on the neuro unit, it came up often—but as a chaplain, I never thought I really needed to know the details. I knew the basics: once brain death is declared, that's the legal time of death. That's when the conversations about donation begin.

Still, something in her tone—a mix of curiosity and invitation—made me say yes.

After observing the brain death testing, I was invited to join the Hospital Development Coordinator during the donation conversation. She gave me simple instructions: *Don't talk about donation. Just be present. If the family brings up anything spiritual, I'll defer to you.* I nodded, humbled to be invited into such a sacred moment.

The conversation went well. The coordinator led with compassion, clarity, and patience. And when the time came, the family said yes.

That donor went on to save three lives through the gift of organ donation—and to enhance the lives of countless others through tissue and eye donation.

What I didn't realize then was that this invitation—this quiet moment in a small ICU conference room—was the beginning of something much bigger. That first "yes" opened the door to many more. It drew me into the work that would eventually become my career: walking alongside families at the intersection of loss and legacy and advocating for the gift of life.

It's been almost eight years since that first donation conversation. Since then, I've been part of hundreds of conversations with grieving families—helping them see how their "yes" can become a silver lining on one of the worst days of their lives.

My career has taken me from the front lines of donation as a Family Services Coordinator, to managing a team of advocates in central Ohio, and now back to the bedside as a donation advocate traveler—spending most of my time in the Appalachian region of the United States.

And yet, in all those conversations, one stands out. One moment when, despite all my training, I broke. I had to excuse myself from the room, find the nearest bathroom, and let the tears come. I'm not someone who cries easily—my Slavic and English roots have taught me how to hold it all in—but this case hit differently.

Thank God I had an orientee with me who was able to carry on the conversation while I pulled myself together. When I returned to the room, I sat beside that man—still grieving, still reeling—and helped him reach a decision that ultimately led to a "yes" for organ donation.

That conversation was the first time I felt the full weight of my calling. The moment where I understood, deep in my bones, why Appalachia matters so much to me. It's the reason my wife and I founded the Whetstone Family Foundation[3]—and the heartbeat behind the stories, research, and reflections that follow in this book.

---

[3] The Whetstone Family Foundation is a charitable organization founded in 2023 to support students in Appalachian Ohio pursuing careers in medicine and the arts. The foundation provides scholarships, mentorship, and advocacy to address educational and

In the first chapter of this book, we'll explore that case in depth. Although it took place after I had already begun researching and developing the training I now offer, it laid the foundation for every story that follows. It reveals why, despite a growing national awareness of organ donation, the unique realities of Appalachia demand a different kind of approach—one shaped not only by science and systems, but by place, people ,and history.

Appalachia is often defined by its geography—mountains, rivers, and winding roads—but the real story lies in its people. As of 2022, more than 26 million Americans call the Appalachian region home, stretching across 13 states from southern New York to northern Mississippi. Despite its beauty and cultural richness, the region carries a disproportionate share of the nation's economic and healthcare burdens.[4]

The median age in Appalachia is 41.3, slightly older than the national average, and its population growth has lagged behind the rest of the country.[5] In rural Appalachian counties, median household incomes fall more than $10,000 below the national rural average.[6] While the region's poverty rate has improved in recent years, it still hovers around 14.3%, with many communities facing persistent financial insecurity.[7]

Educational attainment remains a key challenge and opportunity. Roughly 90% of adults in Appalachia hold a high school diploma, yet only 28% have completed a bachelor's degree.[8]These gaps have long-term

---

financial barriers in underserved rural communities. Learn more at www.whetstonefamilyfoundation.org.

[4] Appalachian Regional Commission. "Appalachia's Population." ARC.gov

[5] ARC. "The Appalachian Region: A Data Overview from the 2017–2021 American Community Survey."

[6] ARC. "Rural Appalachia." ARC.gov

[7] ARC. "ARC Releases New Data Revealing Appalachia's Economic Improvements." ARC.gov

[8] ARC. "Educational Attainment in Appalachia." ARC.gov

implications—not just for economic mobility, but also for access to healthcare, including organ donation education and registration.

Health disparities are particularly acute in this region. Rates of chronic illness are higher, life expectancy is lower, and access to consistent medical care is uneven.[9] These realities—combined with limited infrastructure and lingering mistrust in institutional systems—form the backdrop for every donor conversation in Appalachia. It's not just about medicine; it's about culture, context, and the complex terrain of trust.

---

[9] ARC. "Health Disparities in Appalachia." ARC.gov

CHAPTER ONE

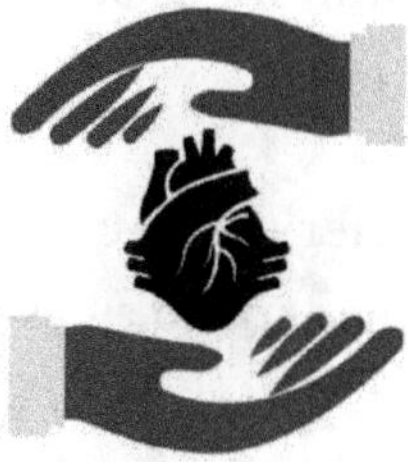

THE ANATOMY OF TRUST

"Nearly 66% of adults in Appalachia read at or below an 8th-grade level."

— Appalachian Learning Initiative

As a healthcare chaplain, I've been trained to walk into intense, emotionally charged situations while keeping my own emotions in check. It's drilled into you early on: *This* isn't *about you. It's about the patient, their family, their grief.* I'm good at this.

I often joke with my counselor that I can flip my emotions on and off like a switch—as the job demands. But in reality, it's not a joke. It's a skill, and it's one I take seriously. Because, when I'm sitting across from a family in the wake of sudden loss, my job isn't to feel my feelings; it's to create a space where they can feel theirs.

This ability has become invaluable in my donation conversations. The capacity to put a family's emotional well-being above my own—to press pause on my own reactions and focus solely on theirs—is how I'm able to do this work and do it well.

I had just started a new traveler contract with an OPO I hadn't worked with before, and they'd assigned me to a case that was on the neuro critical care unit of a hospital I had only been to one time before to help train one of their new hires. The hospital was unfamiliar, the staff mostly strangers, and I was still getting my bearings when the call came in.

My orientee and I arrived just after the day shift had handed off to the night crew. We huddled with the nurse caring for the potential donor—a woman whose husband had just changed her code status to Do Not Resuscitate (DNR). He planned to move her to comfort measures only (CMO) the following day. The gravity of the situation was clear. The prognosis had been accepted. He was ready to say goodbye.

Following protocol, we met with the attending physician to align with the hospital care team and lay the groundwork for our donation conversation. In these moments, it's like standing at the edge of a precipice, knowing that what happens next will forever alter the course of more lives than the ones in that room.

It's in this moment that I remind myself that getting a "yes" from a family means the potential to save eight lives through organ donation. And getting a "no"? It means those same eight people will have to keep waiting.

Sidebar: The Eight Lifesaving Organs

Every organ donor has the potential to save eight lives. It's a number we use often in this work, but what does it really mean?

Heart – Pumps blood and life through the body.

Liver – Filters toxins and produces vital proteins.

Lungs (2) – Two lungs, two recipients.

Pancreas – Regulates blood sugar and insulin production.

Kidneys (2) – Each kidney can go to a different recipient.

Intestines – Essential for nutrient absorption and digestion.

So while there are only six types of organs, there are eight potential gifts because the lungs and kidneys can be divided, doubling their life-saving impact. In some cases, a single recipient may receive more than one organ — such as a heart and kidney, or a liver and pancreas — giving them not just a second chance, but a new beginning through multiple gifts of life.

After we completed our huddle, we asked the nurse to introduce us to the patient's husband. Together, we walked with him to a small family conference room just outside the unit. In those moments, the air is heavy—the weight of what's been said and what's about to be asked hangs between us.

As is custom, I reintroduced myself and the orientee with me. Over the years, I've learned that families in crisis often struggle to retain what they hear in those first few minutes. The shock, the confusion, the sheer emotional overload—it blurs everything. That's why I've made it a practice to repeat myself, to go slowly, to keep my words simple and clear.

I know that when I take my time, when I say things twice if needed, it gives families a moment to catch their breath, to grasp what's happening, and to feel seen amidst the chaos. It's not just about who I am or what I do—it's about giving them the space to take it all in.

"Hi, Jon. Again, my name is Brent. I'm part of the end-of-life care team that works closely with the hospital," I said, keeping my tone steady and calm. "Would you mind telling me a little bit about the conversation you had with Dr. Smith?"

Jon sat there for a moment; his eyes fixed on the table. When he finally spoke, his voice was flat, distant.

"My wife is brain dead," he said.

The words hung in the air. I felt the weight of them—the certainty in his voice, the finality of the phrase. But Jon's wife wasn't brain dead. Not yet. She was missing several of her brainstem reflexes, a serious sign of neurological injury, but it wasn't definitive; there had been no formal testing at this point in her admission. The effects of the medicine that she was on to keep her comfortable could also be masking her true neurological status.

In these moments, the line between clarity and confusion is razor-thin. Families hear phrases like "grave prognosis" or "severe brain injury," and sometimes it all collapses into one phrase: brain dead. But brain death is a specific, clinical diagnosis, with legal and ethical implications—a line that had not yet been crossed.

I stepped out to find the attending, who returned with me to the room. She sat down across from Jon, her expression soft but resolute. With the calm, measured cadence of someone who has delivered such news countless times, she explained that while his wife had suffered a severe anoxic injury, she was not brain dead.

An anoxic brain injury occurs when the brain is completely deprived of oxygen, causing cells to begin dying within minutes. The attending outlined that while there was still some neurological activity, the extentof the damage was severe and could potentially worsen.

"There is still some activity," she said, her voice gentle but firm. "It's possible that she may progress to brain death, or she may remain in a state where the machines are the only things keeping her alive." She reached out, clasping Jon's hand for a brief moment. "I am truly sorry, Jon," she said, before standing and leaving the room.

The words seemed to hang in the air like heavy mist, each syllable weighing Jon down a little further. He nodded mechanically, his eyes fixed on a point somewhere beyond the consult room walls. Then, as if the reality of it all had finally settled over him like a shroud, he looked up.

"Can we… can we just take a break for a moment?" he asked, his voice thin and strained.

My orientee and I rose from our chairs and exited the consult room, Jon trailing behind us. We moved to a small table near the vending machines in the lobby, the fluorescent lights casting a harsh glow over everything. Jon was frantically pressing buttons on his phone, his face tight with frustration. We waited in silence, the hum of the vending machines the only sound.

A few minutes passed, though it felt much longer. Jon's frustration seemed to mount as he repeatedly attempted to call someone. Finally, I stood and walked over to him. "Is everything okay, Jon?"

He looked up, his eyes weary. "I'm trying to get ahold of Stephanie," he said, running a hand through his hair. "She's been up here on and off today and has been with me through all these conversations. It's nice to have someone else here to hear what's being said because... it's all just a bit much."

"I understand, Jon," I said, my tone gentle. "This is a lot to take in, and we're here to help you in any way we can." I took a breath, choosing my words carefully. "First and foremost, I just want to make sure that you understood what the doctor said and to confirm your decision about turning off the machines and allowing your wife to pass naturally."

"That's what she would want," Jon said as he gestured toward his wife's room.

"I just... I don't know what to do. I know she wouldn't want to be hooked up to all those machines. That's not her in there anymore—she's gone. But I never thought she'd be the one to go first. This isn't how it was supposed to be."

This is something I hear often from the spouse left behind. They always expect to be the one who goes first.

I think it's our mind's way of shielding us from the full weight of our mortality—an unconscious hope that we won't have to face life without the person we've built our world around.

But when that moment comes, and they're suddenly gone, there are no words.

Just the quiet, aching realization: you must now walk the rest of your journey without the person you loved most.

"Jon, I know you said this isn't something she would want. Did the two of you ever talk about what she would want—if she ever ended up in a situation like this?"

"Not really," he said quietly.

"That's okay. Most families don't have those conversations—and that's what I'm here for-- to help guide you through this, to talk through some of the next steps, and to walk with you through the decisions that need to be made."

I paused, softening my voice.

"Would you mind if we stepped into the consult room? That way, we'll have a little more privacy as we talk through these sensitive next steps."

"Yeah, we can go back in there," Jon said, as the three of us walked into the consult room and sat across from one another.

"Jon," I began gently, "there are some important next steps we need to talk through."

I paused, ensuring my voice remained calm and steady.

"As I mentioned earlier, I'm part of the end-of-life care team that works closely with the hospital. My role is to meet with families in these difficult moments to talk through decisions that either their loved one has already made—or that they may now be asked to make."

I took a slow breath, keeping my tone even and respectful.

"I represent the Organ Procurement Organization for this state." (Normally, this is where I would share the name of the OPO I work for, but to maintain HIPAA compliance, I'll refer to it simply as 'the OPO' moving forward.)

"We're the organization that works with families like yours," I continued, "and we provide education around organ, tissue, and eye donation."

I leaned in slightly, softening my tone.

"I'm here today because your wife has the rare and unique opportunity to save up to eight lives through the gift of organ donation—and to enhance countless others through tissue donation."

"I'm not sure it's on her license," Jon said, cutting me off.

"It's not, Jon," I replied gently. "That's one of the things I checked before I came in to speak with you. That means *you* have the ability to build a lasting legacy for your wife through the gift of donation."

Jon's eyes darted down as he pulled out his phone, his fingers fumbling with the passcode.

"I just don't know," he said, voice tight. "I need to call Stephanie. Can I call Stephanie?"

"Absolutely, Jon," I said without hesitation. "If you'd like to have Stephanie on the phone, we can absolutely continue this conversation with her as well."

Jon was fumbling with his phone, trying to call. There was no answer.

"I just don't know," he said again, his eyes locked on the screen, avoiding mine.

"Jon," I said gently, "I know this is a lot to take in. We're here to help you through it, and to answer any questions you may have."

He repeated it—quieter this time. "I just don't know."

I gave him a moment. Then, softly:

"Would it be okay if I explained a little bit about the process?"

He looked up, not quite nodding, but not objecting either.

"A lot of families come in with misconceptions about donation," I continued. "They've seen it portrayed on medical dramas and think it plays out that way in real life. But it doesn't. And I've found that when I walk through what the process *actually* looks like, it helps. It clears up the unknowns and makes space for real understanding."

He nodded yes.

I leaned in slightly, speaking with calm and steady rhythm.

"We'll start with some paperwork. That part takes about 45 minutes to an hour. We'll go through a set of medical history questions—that just helps us better understand your wife's health background."

He was still, listening, holding on.

"Once that's complete, my clinical team will begin their process. They'll draw some blood and send it to a specialized facility in Pittsburgh. Jon, that's usually the longest part of everything we do."

I paused to let him catch his breath, then continued.

"That bloodwork helps us in two big ways. First, it checks for any diseases or infections your wife may have had—some things you might not have even known about, but that could affect the safety of donation. And second, we'll get her blood type."

I looked him in the eye.

"Once we have that information back, we can begin finding the people—*the actual individuals*—that your wife can save through her gift of donation."

"I just don't know what to do," Jon said, his voice barely above a whisper.

I nodded, giving him space—and then asked, softly,

"Jon... can I ask something?"

"Yes," he replied, not looking up.

"What is it you're concerned about?"

He shifted slightly, still silent.

"From what you've shared with me about your wife," I continued, "it sounds like you both are the kind of people who give—who show up for others without hesitation. The kind of people who'd give the shirt off their back if someone needed it."

I paused, letting the weight of that truth hang in the air.

"So, I just want to ask—what are you struggling with about donation?"

I didn't want to push too hard. But I could feel it—there was something more underneath his uncertainty.

"I just don't know," he said again, eyes still fixed downward.

Jon, this is a safe space. You can share your concerns with us—no judgment.

Jon began to tear up.

"I don't know how to read," he said quietly. "I really want to do this... but I'm scared. I don't know about the paperwork you talked about. I'm afraid I'm going to sign something I shouldn't be signing."

It hit me like a ton of bricks.

I've sat through countless workshops on health literacy rates in the United States. I've seen the slides, heard the statistics. But I had never seen it so starkly, so personally, as a barrier to donation. Here was a man losing everything, and on top of his grief, he had to worry about us—*about me*—being dishonest. That we might take advantage of his inability to read.

I was flooded with emotion. I don't know if it was because I'd been on the road for a month—away from my wife, away from my kids—or because, in that moment, I truly understood the sacred weight of what it means to meet someone where they are. But for the first time in my professional career, I felt myself beginning to unravel.

In chaplaincy, we're taught a trick when we need to make a quick emotional exit from a patient's room: *fake an injury*. Rub your eye, cough, find some plausible excuse to slip away before the emotion overtakes you.

So I did.

"Jon," I said, trying to hold my composure, "I have an idea. I'll be right back."

I turned quickly and left the room—leaving my orientee behind, no doubt confused—and made a beeline for the men's room. I needed a moment. Not to hide, but to feel. To breathe. To pray.

I pushed through the door of the men's room and let it close behind me. My legs were shaking. I didn't make it far.

I leaned against the cold tile wall, and before I knew it, I was sliding down, shoulders trembling, tears finally breaking loose. There wasn't time to think, to rationalize, to perform. The weight of it all—Jon's fear, his honesty, his vulnerability—collapsed on top of me like a flood.

I sobbed. Quietly, but uncontrollably. I don't think I had ever wept like that in a hospital. Not as a professional. Not in uniform. But in that moment, I wasn't the professional. I was just *me*—a husband missing his family, a father thinking about what it would be like to lose a child, a man of faith suddenly overwhelmed by the sacredness of trust.

All Jon wanted was to do the right thing. To say yes to donation. To honor his loved one. But he was scared. Not because he didn't care—but because he couldn't read. Because he was afraid someone like me would take advantage of that. And that broke me.

This wasn't just about literacy. This was about dignity. About how the systems we work in—no matter how well-intentioned—can still create fear in the hearts of the grieving.

And for the first time, I saw it clearly: *meeting people where they are isn't a technique—it's an act of reverence.*

There on that bathroom floor, still in my scrubs, I prayed without words. I asked for the strength to return to Jon not as someone with answers, but as someone worthy of the trust he had just extended.

Eventually, I stood up, wiped my eyes, and looked in the mirror. I didn't need to hide what had happened. I just needed to carry it with me.

Because chaplaincy doesn't call us to be unshakable. It calls us to be present.

And I was going back into that room to do just that.

I walked back into the room, still carrying the weight of what had just happened—but steadied now by purpose.

Jon looked up, eyes searching mine. He didn't need words to ask if I had figured something out.

And I had.

"Jon," I said gently, "I know how we can move forward in a way that feels safe for you. I'd like to bring in the hospital chaplain. Not someone from my team, but a neutral third party—someone who isn't connected to the donation process. They can sit with us, listen to everything I explain, and help make sure that what you're agreeing to is exactly what's written down. No tricks. No fine print. Just truth."

He nodded, slowly at first, then with more conviction. I could see the fear begin to lift. He didn't want someone to do it *for* him—he just wanted to know he wasn't alone. That someone was standing beside him, not above him. That someone would bear witness.

Calling the chaplain wasn't a formality. It was an act of *restoration*. It returned agency to a man who'd had everything else stripped away—his wife, his plans, his certainty. And now, it gave him the confidence to say *yes* to something brave and selfless, without the fear of being betrayed by the fine print.

This wasn't just about verifying a document. It was about honoring a man's courage with transparency and trust.

And I knew in my bones: this is what it means to advocate—not to speak for someone, but to *stand with them*, exactly where they are.

I was so grateful when the chaplain arrived.

They were an older Episcopal priest—seasoned, calm, and quietly present in the way only a long-time chaplain can be. They worked part-time at the hospital but carried themselves with the steady gravity of someone who had spent a lifetime holding sacred space. And, most importantly, they spoke my language—not just the theological vocabulary, but the unspoken rhythms of chaplaincy. The reading of rooms. The holding of breath. The weight of silence.

They could see it in me right away.

Not just the emotion I was trying to keep tucked beneath the surface, but the burden I carried—the deep concern I had for Jon, the care I was taking to protect his dignity, the sacred tension between my professional responsibility and my very human ache.

We didn't need to say much. That's the beauty of this work when it's done well. Sometimes presence is the most fluent language we have.

The chaplain nodded, gently took a seat beside Jon, and simply said, "I'm here to support you in whatever way you need. Let's walk through this together."

And in that moment, the room changed. The fear softened. The air settled. And I knew—we had found the way forward.

Jon looked at the chaplain, then at me. You could see it in his eyes—he was still grieving, still unsure of so much. But now, he wasn't alone in that space. He was surrounded by people who weren't pressuring him, but honoring him.

We went through the paperwork slowly, carefully. I read each section aloud, pausing after every paragraph to check for understanding. The chaplain listened, offered clarifications when needed, and affirmed that everything we discussed was reflected on the page.

Jon asked a few questions—simple, direct, brave questions. And when we reached the final section, he looked up and said, "I want to do this. For her."

With his signature, everything shifted.

It wasn't just ink on a page. It was a sacred act of trust. Of courage. Of love. And I knew what a miracle it was that we had reached this moment—not because of my skills, or a textbook protocol, but because we met Jon with honesty, humility, and human presence.

He said *yes*—not because we convinced him, but because he was seen, respected, and supported.

That's the anatomy of a yes. It's not a transaction. It's a relationship. A moment of transformation built on the fragile trust between grief and grace.

And as I watched him press pen to paper, I knew: I had never been more humbled to bear witness.

Jon pressed the pen to the paper slowly, with steady hands but trembling breath. There was no fanfare, no applause—just the quiet gravity of a man doing right by his wife, even when the path forward felt uncertain.

When he finished signing, he looked at me. There were no words exchanged—just a nod. But it was one I will never forget. It carried the weight of trust, of relief, of something holy.

The chaplain offered a simple blessing—nothing scripted, just a few heartfelt words of comfort—and placed a gentle hand on Jon's shoulder. I thanked them quietly, knowing their presence had made the impossible possible.

We collected the paperwork, answered Jon's last questions, and left him in peace.

Outside the room, I stood in the hallway for a moment. I didn't move. I didn't speak. I just let it all settle—the emotion, the sacredness, the responsibility. I had been trained to guide families through this process. I had been certified, evaluated, and mentored. But nothing in my training had prepared me for the spiritual weight of that "yes."

We talk often about *informed consent* in healthcare. We define it in legal terms, in procedural steps, in best practices. But we rarely talk about what it feels like—what it *means*—to give someone the dignity of understanding. Of safety. Of being known.

Jon's fear wasn't rooted in skepticism of donation. It was rooted in a deeper, more human fear: that he would be taken advantage of in his most vulnerable hour. That his inability to read might be used against him. That the system would fail to meet him where he was.

That moment changed me.

It taught me that the real work of an advocate—especially in the world of organ donation—is not about persuasion. It's about *presence*. It's about giving people the time, space, and trust they need to make a sacred decision with clarity and peace.

Yes, we need paperwork. Yes, we need signatures. But more than that, we need to bring integrity into the room.

Jon didn't say yes because I convinced him. He said yes because, in that moment, he felt safe. He felt seen. And he believed—deeply—that his wife's life could mean something beyond her death.

That's the kind of "yes" that stays with you. Not in the checkboxes or the consent forms, but in your spirit. And it's the kind of "yes" I carry with me every time I walk into another hospital room, unsure of what I'll face—but certain of the sacred ground I stand on.

Health Literacy & Organ Donation: The Hidden Barrier

Only 12% of U.S. adults have *proficient* health literacy.[10]

Nearly 9 out of 10 adults struggle to understand and use everyday health information that is routinely available in health care facilities, media, and communities.[11]

Individuals with limited health literacy are less likely to:

Understand complex medical terms (e.g., "neurological death" vs. "brain death")

Comprehend consent forms or risk-benefit explanations

Ask clarifying questions out of fear of judgment

Limited literacy is correlated with lower rates of organ donor registration, particularly in underserved and rural communities, where institutional distrust may already be high.(Source: Journal of Health Communication, 2016)

In donation conversations, reading level mismatches are common. A 2019 study found that most donor authorization forms are written at a 12th-

---

[10] National Assessment of Adult Literacy, 2003

[11] Source: U.S. Department of Health and Human Services

grade reading level, while the average U.S. adult reads at a 7th–8th grade level.

Language and literacy barriers are identified as a top non-medical deterrent to organ donation in hospitals and community-based donation initiatives.

CHAPTER TWO

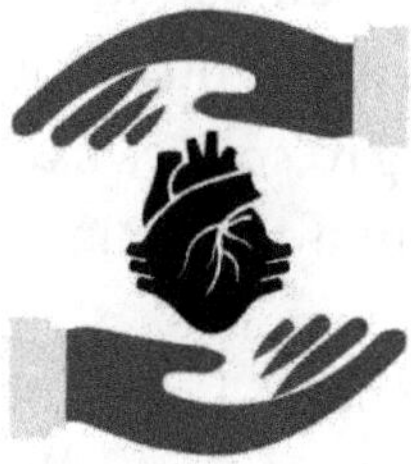

THE ANATOMY OF SILENCE

"In many Appalachian communities, silence is not avoidance—
it's how pain is carried with dignity."

— Appalachian Regional Studies Journal

Nearly a decade ago—though it feels like a lifetime now—I took my first hesitant steps into the world of chaplaincy by enrolling in a unit of Clinical Pastoral Education. CPE, as it's called, is a form of professional ministry training that drops students into real-world clinical environments and asks them to reflect deeply on their encounters, growing through supervised experience.

I didn't want to be there. I walked in convinced I already knew what ministry was. I had preached sermons, sat at hospital bedsides, prayed with grieving families. What more could they possibly teach me?

That arrogance made my first unit a struggle. I butted heads with my supervisor more times than I can count. She had this way of calling me out—not unkindly, but directly. "You go into fix-it mode," she'd say after a patient visit. "You're trying to solve what can't be solved. You need to stop talking so much. Get comfortable in the silence."

"Get comfortable in the silence." I remember thinking, *What on earth is that supposed to mean?* At the time, it sounded more like a fortune cookie than a clinical insight.

But years later, I'd come to understand exactly what she meant. In the sacred space between life and death, between hope and letting go, silence is often where the truth begins to speak. And as I stood with families facing impossible decisions about organ donation, it was that silence—not words—that held the most grace.

Silence, in that sacred moment, was exactly what was needed—giving space for a family to let go, so their father and husband could go on to restore sight through eye donation and bring healing to countless others through the gift of tissue.

It was a sweltering summer afternoon when my AOC, or Administrator on Call, reached out. I was dispatched immediately for what we call a HOT approach. In our world, HOT stands for "Hand on Tube"—a signal that the family is at the bedside, preparing to withdraw life support, and that a donation conversation needs to happen without delay.

HOT approaches don't leave much room for preparation. There's no time to comb through the EMR—the electronic medical record—to piece together what happened or who this person was. You go in blind, your only focus: the family in front of you.

Thirty minutes later, I walked onto the unit and found the primary nurse. Before anything else, we always huddle with the care team—usually the nurse and attending physician—to align our approach. It's not just about medical facts; it's about presence, tone, and trust. We walk together so the family doesn't feel like they're walking alone.

In that huddle, I learned that the patient—a father—had died from an accidental overdose. His youngest daughter had handed him what she believed was a simple pain pill. It turned out to be laced with fentanyl.

The nurse pulled me aside before I could even approach the room. She let me know, in no uncertain terms, that the patient's wife and son were extremely upset—and that any mention of donation would not be well received. "You may want to just let them withdraw," she said gently, clearly trying to protect the family from more pain.

I nodded, thanked her for the insight, and reassured her that I would be careful—gentle. Nurses often become fierce guardians of the families they've cared for day after day, and I've learned to respect that deeply. But I've also learned something else: it's not always that they're opposed to donation. Sometimes it's that they've seen the family endure so much already, and the idea of one more conversation—especially one this emotionally charged—feels like too much.

But what we offer isn't just another conversation. It's the possibility of meaning inside the chaos. It's a sliver of light in the dark. It's legacy. And while these discussions can feel impossibly heavy in the moment, I've seen time and time again how, months or even years later, families will reach back out—not in anger, but in gratitude. Gratitude for the chance to say yes. Gratitude that their loved one was able to live on through organ, tissue, and eye donation.

As I entered the room, I saw them—two people, both broken, exhausted, and angry. I paused at the door, gently knocked, and asked for permission to enter their sacred space. "Come in," they said.

I stepped inside, moved a chair across the room, and sat down at a respectful distance. "My name is Brent," I began softly. "I'm here to help walk you through some of the options you have for next steps. But before we begin—would you mind sharing your names and how you're related to Ricky?"

"I'm Carol," she said. "Ricky's wife. And this is our son, Blake."

Blake looked like he hadn't slept in days—his eyes heavy, his body sagging under the weight of grief. Still, he sat upright, trying to be strong for his mother, even as tears lingered just beneath the surface.

"Again, my name is Brent," I said gently, "and I just want to say how truly sorry I am to be meeting you under these circumstances. Typically, I have a bit of time to review a patient's chart before sitting down with family, but in this case, I wasn't able to do that. Would you mind sharing with me what brought Ricky here?"

Carol didn't hesitate.

"Morgan," she said sharply. "Morgan is what brought him here. We told her these goddamned drugs were going to catch up to her eventually—we just never expected *her dad* to be the one who overdosed. He's been sober for 20 years. Ever since the kids were born. That's why he couldn't handle the fentanyl."

My heart dropped. "Oh no… I'm so sorry."

"It's not your fault," Carol replied, waving off my apology. Then her face hardened. "Morgan just better hope the police find her before I do."

"Mom..." Blake said quietly, his voice strained.

He glanced toward me, as if suddenly remembering I was still there. The room was thick with anger, pain, and the unbearable irony of a father's overdose linked to the very daughter he'd stayed sober for. There was no easy path through this moment—only presence.

"A few days ago, me and Dad were working on the deck," Blake said, his voice tight. "We were expanding it, and he did too much. Hurt his back. Morgan decided this week she was going to be back in our lives, and she was at home. She heard him say his back hurt, and she... she gave him one of her pain pills."

He paused. The anger rose like heat.

"Now he's dead. She fucking killed our dad, man. And now she's on the run. The cops are looking for her."

"I can't even begin to imagine what you're going through," I said softly.

"They'll get her," Carol muttered, holding her stare on the wall. "We've got Ring cameras at the house. She's got one at her apartment too. As soon as she shows up, we'll know."

Silence fell over the room. Long. Heavy. Sacred. We sat in it together. No words could touch the depth of what had just been said.

But I also knew that silence sometimes opens the door for something else—something redemptive.

Gently, I turned to Blake. "Blake, I heard you say earlier that your dad is dead. Would you mind sharing with me what Dr. Kline told you?"

Blake looked down at the floor. "Dr. Kline said Dad wasn't going to recover, technically—that he'd still be alive—but he'd be on a ventilator for the rest of his life. It's not living. It's surviving. And Dad always said he never wanted that."

Carol nodded quietly in agreement.

"That's what Dr. Kline told me as well," I said quietly. "And I'm just so sorry. So sorry that you all are having to go through this. Sometimes... life just isn't fair."

We sat there in silence for a few moments—each person wrapped in their own thoughts, each holding their grief in a different way. I didn't rush to fill the quiet. Sometimes presence speaks louder than words.

After a while, Carol broke the stillness. "What happens now?"

I turned to her gently. "Well Carol, if I'm understanding what you said earlier—that Ricky wouldn't want to live like this—then there's an important decision ahead. And from what you've shared with me, it sounds like Ricky was the kind of man who gave without hesitation. You told me he was helping Blake when he got hurt. He just strikes me as someone who'd give the shirt off his back if he saw someone in need."

Carol nodded slowly. "He really was. There was this one time—we were driving down the road in the rain, and Ricky saw a young man walking. He pulled over to give him a ride. I asked him what he was doing—'this could be an axe murderer!' I said—but he just looked at me and said, 'He looked like he needed help.' That's who Ricky was. He just... helped."

"Well," I said gently, "I'm here to ask if Ricky might be willing to help—just one more time. In addition to supporting you through these next steps, I have the privilege of sharing how Ricky's legacy could live on through others… through the life-saving gift of organ, tissue, and eye donation."

"Yes!" Blake said without hesitation, his voice firm and clear. "Dad would want to do that. If he knew he could save lives, he'd do it in a heartbeat."

Carol nodded slowly, tears rising in her eyes. "He really would," she whispered, her voice catching.

"Thank you, Blake," I said, humbled by the clarity of his response. "Would it be okay if I explained a little about what that process looks like?"

They both nodded.

And just like that, the room shifted—not away from grief, but into something sacred. A space where loss and generosity could coexist. Where goodbye could also mean giving life.

As I began to explain the process—what would happen next, what donation would mean for Ricky and for others—I saw something shift in Carol's expression. It was subtle at first: a tightening around the eyes, a slow intake of breath. The look of realization. Not resistance or fear, but the quiet dawning that organ donation was a process. A real one. One with steps, timelines, and decisions. It was something she had been willing to say yes to in spirit—but now that it was real, she carried questions. Questions she may not have even known she had.

And that's the thing. Most people never find themselves in this place. Only about 3 in every 1,000 deaths occur in a way that makes organ donation medically possible.[12] That means very few families ever walk this road—fewer still with any prior understanding of what lies ahead. The rarity of the moment doesn't make it any less sacred, but it does mean that many families are asked to navigate the most significant decision of their lives in a space they never expected to be. And so, in those moments, it becomes our job not just to explain—but to sit, to honor, and to walk alongside them with grace.

So that's what I did. I walked them through the ins and outs of the donation process—each step, each detail—careful not to overwhelm, but knowing it was already a lot. At one point, I paused and said, "I know this is a tremendous amount of information to take in. In just a few short hours, you've experienced every emotion imaginable—shock, sorrow, uncertainty—and now you're being asked to absorb complex medical and logistical information while still trying to grieve." I looked at them and added, "I'm sorry for that. I wish there were a gentler way to do this. But I want you to know I'm here. To walk with you through this, to answer your questions, and to be your support—for as long as you need me."

"I just don't know," Carol said quietly.

They're words I never want to hear—especially after a family has already agreed to donation. My mind began to race. Had I said something wrong? Was there a detail that shifted their decision? I felt the familiar tug of self-doubt begin to creep in.

"What questions do you have, Carol?" I asked gently.

---

[12] U.S. Department of Health & Human Services. "Organ Donation Statistics." *organdonor.gov*. https://www.organdonor.gov/learn/organ-donation-statistics

She glanced at Blake, who looked down at the floor. They both did. The silence settled in, thick but necessary. My instinct was to start talking, to fill the space with reassurance or explanation—but I resisted. This wasn't about me. This was their time. Their moment to grieve, to pause, to sit with the weight of what was being asked. To decide if they were still ready to walk this path.

We sat together in that quiet for a few more moments.

"I've been doing this a long time," I finally said. "And honestly, most families don't know what questions to ask. One of the most common things I hear is, 'What if I can't afford this?' And that's such an important question. What many families don't realize is that donation comes at no cost to them. Once we complete the paperwork, my organization covers everything that happens from that point until the recovery is complete."

"Oh, that's good," Carol said, exhaling just slightly. "I was worried about that."

She paused again. "I just think… we need to pull the tubes now."

"Carol, I completely understand," I said. "If that's what you feel is best, I can let Dr. Kline know that's the decision. I'm here to support you, no matter what you choose."

But something in my gut told me not to leave. Not yet.

I could see it—something unspoken hanging in the air. The way Carol and Blake kept glancing at each other, then back down at the floor, as if wrestling with a question they didn't want to voice. There was a tension there. Not resistance, but hesitation. Almost embarrassment.

And then I did what I often do in those moments: I mentally scanned through every family I've ever sat with. Faces. Names. Tears. Questions.

They all flashed through my mind, like a silent roll call of memory. What was I missing?

My role is to walk families through this process—to educate, support, and honor the gift of life through donation. But in this moment, I felt like I was overlooking something important. I knew they wanted to honor Ricky's legacy. They told me that. I also remembered that Ricky was the sole provider. Carol had mentioned she hadn't worked in years.

And then it struck me.

"You know," I said gently, "when my dad died two years ago, it was completely unexpected. I was on my way to the hospital to talk to a family about donation when my phone rang. It was my mom. I almost sent it to voicemail—I was trying to get out the door—but it was Mom, so I answered.

"I think Dad isn't breathing," she said, almost as soon as I picked up.

"I told her to call 911" and said "I'd be right there."

"In those moments, everything just… paused. And one of the first things I remember thinking—after the shock—was, *How am I going to pay for the funeral?* Dad didn't have insurance. There was no plan. No safety net. Just grief, and the weight of what comes next."

I looked at them both. "If you're anything like we were—and like so many of the families I work with—that might be what's sitting in the back of your mind right now. Not just grief. But the unknown. *How the heck are we going to afford what comes next?*"

Carol burst into tears. "Brent, I just don't know how we're going to pay for it," she said, her voice cracking under the weight of it all. "This is all Morgan's fault. I've lost everything."

Blake stood and wrapped his arms around her. "Mom, Dad would want us to say yes," he said quietly.

"I know, Blakey," she replied, resting her head against his shoulder. "I know he would."

I waited a moment, allowing them that space, then gently spoke. "Carol," I said, "can I share something I often tell families about our process?"

She nodded through her tears. "Yes."

"Donation is a process," I began. "And it takes time. But I always tell families—don't wish that time away. This process gives you something incredibly important right now: *a pause*. Time to breathe. Time to rest. Time to begin figuring out what comes next."

I leaned in just a bit, keeping my voice steady. "You'll be able to go home and call your friends, your family. You can tell them that Ricky has the potential to save lives—that he's going to be a donor hero. And knowing the kind of man Ricky was, how quick he was to help anyone in need, I imagine you're going to have people who are ready to return that kindness. People who will want to stand by you."

She listened, tears still in her eyes, but her shoulders softened just slightly.

"Use this time, Carol," I said. "Use it to rest. To make calls. To begin planning, to start figuring out the next steps—without having to do it all right now. We'll walk through this together."

"Let's do it," she said.

We signed the paperwork, and shortly after, Carol and Blake went home. A few days later, I returned to the hospital to support the honor walk and the final moments of extubation.

When I arrived, the unit was full—overflowing with people. Family. Friends. Neighbors. Some I recognized; many I didn't. All of them gathered in quiet reverence, wearing matching shirts that read *Justice for Ricky*.

I found Carol and Blake standing off to the side.

"Quite the impressive turnout," I said softly.

Carol nodded, her eyes scanning the room. "I told you," she replied. "He helped a lot of people. Everyone here has a story to tell—every single one of them. Ricky made sure of it."

I smiled. "Well, I have something I'd like to present to you. I think it would be a fitting way to honor Ricky—and give everyone here a chance to show him just how much he meant."

We gathered the group in the waiting room, and I presented Carol and Blake with the *Donor Hero Medal*, a token of recognition we give to families on behalf of their loved ones who choose to give the gift of life. Then, with the room quiet and full of emotion, I read the *Moment of Honor*—the reflection we share before a recovery begins, a moment set aside to honor the donor's life and legacy.

In the time leading up to extubation, one by one, people came to me—friends, coworkers, neighbors. Each with a story. A ride given. A bill paid. Groceries dropped off without being asked. Gas money slipped into someone's hand when times were tight. Over and over, I heard the same phrase: *Ricky just showed up. Every time.*

And so it was no surprise to anyone that he showed up one final time.

Although Ricky did not pass within the medical window needed for organ donation, he still gave the gift of sight to someone in need through eye donation. He will also help countless others through tissue donation.

His legacy lives not only in the lives he saved—but in the community he built. A community that showed up for him, just as he had shown up for them.

In Appalachia, loss wears many faces—but few have cut as deeply as the quiet devastation of overdose. It's not just a crisis. It's a wound that doesn't scab. A mother who gets the call too soon. A grandmother raising a second generation. A town that learns to count eulogies by season.

Somewhere along the ridge lines and river valleys, death from overdose became less of an exception and more of a drumbeat. In 2020 alone, more than 7,000 lives were lost to opioid-related overdoses across the Appalachian region, accounting for over three-fourths of all drug fatalities that year[13]. That year, Appalachia's overdose death rate was 50% higher than the national average[14]—a gap that continues to widen.

To put it plainly: if you live in rural Appalachia, you are significantly more likely to die from an overdose than your peers elsewhere. Recent studies show opioid overdose mortality rates 72% higher in Appalachian counties compared to non-Appalachian ones[15]. Among adults aged 25–54, that

---

[13] Appalachian Regional Commission. *Appalachian Diseases of Despair Update: November 2022.* https://w ww.arc.gov

[14] Appalachian Health Data: Opioid Misuse. *Health in Appalachia.* https://healthinappalachia.org/issue-briefs/opioid-misuse

[15] National Association of Counties. *How Appalachian Counties Can Combat the Opioid Epidemic.* https://w ww.naco.org/resources/press/new -report-outlines-how-appalachian-counties-can-do-more-less-combat-opioid-epidemic

disparity reaches 64%[16]. These aren't abstract numbers. They are lived realities—felt in funeral homes, empty chairs at Thanksgiving, and children left behind.

Between 2018 and 2021, the opioid-related death rate in rural Appalachian counties rose from 0.43 to 0.62 deaths per 1,000 residents[17]. And still, the region's resources remain strained—its caregivers and advocates often operating without the institutional scaffolding afforded to more urban areas.

In these moments—these quiet, devastating losses—families are sometimes presented with a singular and sacred opportunity: the chance to say yes. The chance to allow legacy to take root in the very soil that grief has broken open. And for those of us who do this work, understanding the weight of Appalachian overdose is not just context. It is call.

---

16 Appalachian Regional Commission. *Addressing Substance Abuse in Appalachia.* https://w ww.arc.gov/addressing-substance-abuse-i n-appalachia

17 Franzosa, Emily et al. "Community-Based Strategies to Address Opioid Use in Rural Appalachia." *J Health Care Poor Underserved.* 2023;34(1):47–65. https://pmc.ncbi.nlm.nih.gov/articles/PMC10349683

CHAPTER THREE

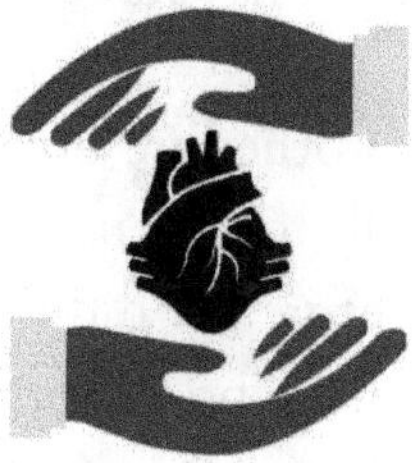

THE ANATOMY OF A SUPERHERO

"We can't all be heroes, because somebody has to sit on the curb and clap as they go by."

— Will Rogers

I am the son and brother of addicts.

That's not a sentence that came easily. In fact, I didn't say it aloud until my Clinical Pastoral Education—when the vulnerability was required, and the silence no longer served me. I think most of us carry the instinct to protect the image of a perfect life. But addiction has no respect for appearances. Like so many other families, mine has felt the long shadow of this disease.

Because of that, every time I sit with a donor family who has just lost someone to addiction, I see my own reflection in their grief. I think—this could have been me. This could have been us.

Thankfully, my mother and brother are both in recovery now—six years clean and counting. But not all stories end that way. My father's didn't. As I mentioned in the chapter before, he didn't die of an overdose. He died of a heart attack at 62 years old—no history of heart disease, no warning signs. Just a body that had carried too much for too long. Years of drug use had worn him down from the inside out.

His death wasn't sudden in the medical sense, but in every other way, it caught us off guard. Addiction stole him by inches.

And so, when I show up for these families—when I walk into a room where overdose is the villain—I'm not just there as a Donation Advocate. I'm there as a witness. A son. A brother. Someone who knows that behind every "yes" to donation is a lifetime of complexity, struggle, and the kind of courage that doesn't always get seen.

Every donor—and every donor family—holds a sacred place in my heart. I remember them often, sometimes in flashes, sometimes in quiet prayers. Each one is unique. Each name a story. And behind every "yes" to donation is a story of loss—often sudden, often tragic.

But there are some that stay with me longer.

Some families leave more than memories. They leave a weight. A grief that doesn't quite lift. These are the ones that hit too close to home. The ones where I see my own family in their faces. The ones where I don't just walk with them through their loss—I carry it, too. Not because I have to, but because something in that moment broke me open, and I never quite closed the same way again.

This was such a donor.

I had never been on a pediatric burn unit before. In fact, I had never been on a burn unit at all, so I wasn't quite sure what to expect. The air was heavy with antiseptic and sorrow, and everything felt quieter than it should have—like even the walls knew not to make a sound. The lights were dimmed, but nothing could soften the reality of the place. Tiny beds. Tiny bodies. The kind of suffering that feels unjust simply because of how small and innocent it is.

The smell is something that sticks with me.

Not in the way most people think—burned flesh. It was more complex than that. It was the smell of clinging smoke. Something that smelled like pain: like trauma lingering in the air long after the flames were gone. I can still recall it when I walk into certain rooms or when the temperature in the air changes just right. It sneaks up on me, uninvited and unforgotten.

That smell was the first thing to greet me when I stepped onto the unit, and it was the last thing to leave when I walked out.

I stopped at the nurses' station to check in. This was my first day on this particular case. I hadn't been the one to authorize donation, nor had I been present for those first impossible conversations. I was there to relieve my colleague—who had finally gone home after nearly twenty-four hours at the hospital, standing watch, walking with the family through every step of the pain. She had been their anchor, and now I was stepping into the space she had held with care and exhaustion. It's always delicate, that handoff. You're not just picking up paperwork—you're stepping into someone else's grief mid-chapter, hoping you can read the tone well enough not to fumble the next lines.

I introduced myself and got report from the bedside nurse. The family had stepped off the unit to get some fresh air—a momentary reprieve from the weight they'd been carrying for days. I used the time to quietly step into the room and meet the donor. He was thirteen. The same age as my son at the time. And the resemblance was unnerving. Same tousled hair, same lanky frame caught somewhere between childhood and adolescence. When I looked at him, I didn't see a stranger—I saw my boy. And just like that, the walls between professional and personal blurred. Thirteen years old, with his whole life ahead of him… gone in an instant, lost to a house fire that raged faster than anyone could have predicted. Life is just not fair sometimes.

One of the questions I'm asked most often as a chaplain is this: Why does God allow bad things to happen to good people? To children? The training tells us to respond with another question—*What do you think?*—so as not to project our beliefs. But the truth is, I don't know. I wish I did. I wish I had something more comforting than silence to offer in moments like these. Some theological framework that could make it make sense. But sometimes the most honest thing I can do is simply sit in the mystery with them, with you—and whisper with all the faith I can muster: *God is here, too.*

After spending a few quiet moments at the bedside, I stepped back out into the hallway and returned to the nurses' station. The weight of the room lingered in my chest, but there was still work to be done. I needed to chart my presence, document the report I'd received from the bedside nurse, and get caught up on the case. I opened the electronic medical record and began reading through the earlier notes—each line a window into the slow, painful unraveling of a family's world. I searched for news articles too, trying to piece together the story behind the tragedy. A fire. A rescue. A community shaken. I wasn't there when they arrived, but now I was part of it—folded into this family's unimaginable loss.

It was our policy to remain on-site around the clock for all pediatric donors, to ensure a consistent presence and emotional support for both the family and the care team. That meant long nights in hospitals not built for rest, in units filled with impossibly small beds and heartbreakingly large grief. I settled in, knowing that tonight would be less about action and more about presence. Not fixing. Not leading. Just being—so that when the family returned, they would not return to silence, but to someone ready to walk with them through the hardest night of their lives.

A few hours had passed, and I realized I hadn't seen the family. I returned to the patient's room—empty. I checked the family waiting area—also empty. A subtle unease settled in. *Where were they?* I thought to myself. It felt odd, the absence. As I walked back toward the nurses' station, I noticed campus police standing nearby, chatting with staff. They were talking about my donor—his case, the fire, the aftermath. I approached, mentioned that I hadn't yet had a chance to meet the parents. One of the officers shrugged, and, with a smirk, said, "They're probably doped out in the parking deck somewhere."

His tone was casual, dismissive. "Oh?" I said, my voice steady but curious. "Yeah," he continued, "they were passed out high as kites yesterday in the parking garage, so I'm sure that's where they are now."

I felt my jaw tighten. I wanted to snap. I've learned—often the hard way—that this kind of cynicism is a defense mechanism. It's what people do in healthcare when the weight of it all becomes too much. A symptom of caregiver fatigue, not malice. Still, it cut deep. These were grieving parents—parents who had just lost their child. I took a breath, steadied myself, and responded gently. "I hear you," I said, "but let's remember... if I had just lost my child, I might be looking for a way to numb the pain, too. They're not okay. None of us would be. Instead of speculating, maybe we can try to show them some compassion—support them through the hell they're walking through right now."

It wasn't about defending addiction or dismissing the realities that come with it. It was about dignity. About remembering that no matter what brought them here, they were still someone's mom, someone's dad, and their son was still a donor hero.

At that moment, Bobby and Jenny—both in their late twenties—appeared at the nurses' station. These were Adam's parents. They looked exhausted, like people who had been through hell and still had more to endure. I quickly stood and stepped toward them.

"My name is Brent," I said gently. "I'm the Family Services Coordinator who will be with you tonight. Why don't we step into the family conference room, so I can give you an update on where we are in the process?"

The truth was, I didn't have any new information to share, but I wanted to spare them from sensing the uncomfortable conversation that had just taken place at the nurses' station. In that moment, my role was to shield them from any further harm—or judgment.

We walked down the long, sterile hallway—each step taking us closer to Adam's room and further from the nurses' station. The family conference room wasn't like the stark, clinical spaces found elsewhere in the hospital. This one had families in mind. Couches lined the walls, a small play area waited in the corner for children who needed distraction during the hardest conversations of their lives, and a circle of rocking chairs sat ready, inviting closeness.

We settled into that circle. Bobby stared off into the distance, still locked in shock. Jenny's eyes were rimmed with tears, but she held herself stiff, trying to be strong.

"I'm so sorry," I said quietly.

"Why did this have to happen to us— to Adam? He didn't deserve this," Jenny's voice trembled. "I fell asleep while he was gaming... he must have gone to bed on his own, because they found him under his bed."

"I'm sorry, Jenny. I can't even imagine."

"It should have been me," she whispered.

Don't say that, Jenny," Bobby said softly, breaking his silence. "It's not your fault."

"If I hadn't gone to bed early, maybe this wouldn't have happened," she snapped back, the grief in her voice sharper than she intended.

I leaned in gently, cutting through the heavy air. "Do they know what happened?" I asked, giving her a lifeline away from self-blame—an opening to shift the focus from guilt to understanding.

"It was about 9:30," Jenny began, her voice trembling. "I had just worked a double at the restaurant, and I was exhausted. Bobby was still at work, and I told Adam I was going to bed. I took a quick shower, but it completely wore me out, so I lay down.

The next thing I remember was waking to the sound of sirens in the distance and someone pounding on our door. A woman driving by saw flames shooting out of the top of the house and stopped. If she hadn't... I wouldn't be sitting here right now.

When I woke up, my room was filled with smoke. I ran to my door, but it was surrounded by fire. I had to get to Adam. I crawled out my window—cut myself on the way down—" She glanced at her arms, the fresh cuts and bruised hands telling their own story.

"I ran around to the side of the house where Adam's room is, pounding on the wall to wake him. He sleeps upstairs. I must have woken him because I saw him come to the window. He was trying to get it open, but he couldn't. I was jumping, climbing on anything I could, trying to get to my baby boy. But I couldn't.

I ran to the front door, but it was locked. I couldn't get back into my room to grab the keys in the kitchen. I pushed, I kicked, I threw myself against it, but it wouldn't budge. The lady was on the phone with 911. The police arrived first and kicked the door down, but the fire was too much. The firefighters came minutes later. They found Adam hiding under his bed. My poor baby. I couldn't get to him."

"He had to be so scared," Jenny whispered, her voice breaking. "He crawled under his bed to hide… and he was all alone. I'm his mother—I should have gotten to him."

Bobby reached over, trying to place a comforting hand on her knee, but she pulled away, her grief too sharp to touch. She stood, her eyes fixed on some point far away.

"All I can see," she continued, her voice cracking, "is my baby standing in the window, looking out at me. I'm supposed to protect him… and I didn't."

I felt that familiar tightening in the back of my throat—the one that comes when you're fighting back tears. All I could picture was this mother, frantic and desperate, trying to save her only child. I imagined her pounding on the walls, calling his name, while he stood there in the window—trapped, terrified, and unable to reach her. My only hope was that, in those final moments, he knew she was there. That he felt her love in the fight she waged to get to him.

I took a deep breath and reminded myself—this isn't about me. It's about them. My role is to stand in this storm with them, to help them navigate their grief without trying to steer it somewhere it doesn't want to go. Jenny needed someone who could sit in her pain without looking away, without trying to fix it. Bobby needed someone to steady the room when the weight of it all threatened to pull them both under. I leaned forward, closing the space between us.

"Jenny," I said quietly, "you fought for him with everything you had. That matters."

Her shoulders softened just enough to let a sliver of light through the heavy armor of guilt she was carrying. Bobby reached for her hand again, and this time she let him. We stayed in the silence—not to patch it over, but to honor it.

"I don't know why this happened," she whispered.

"Jenny," I said, "I wish there were words that could take this pain from you and Bobby—but there aren't. Nothing I say will erase what you're walking through right now. It's not natural for parents to lose their children. It's not supposed to happen this way. I don't know your whole story, but from the time I've spent with you, I can see it—you both loved Adam deeply, and you are both stronger than you realize. It takes a great deal of strength to say yes to donation."

"It's what Adam would have wanted," Bobby said. "He loved Superman—he was always playing superheroes. The idea that he could go on to save someone else's life... that's exactly what our boy would have wanted."

And that's exactly what Adam did. Because his parents were willing to say yes to donation, their son lives on in three people—becoming the superhero he had always dreamed of being.

That was the only time I ever met Bobby and Jenny. I don't know how their story has unfolded in the years since that night. My hope is that, even in the shadow of losing their son, they have held on to the truth that he gave the gift of life to others—and that this became a source of strength, a reason to keep moving forward.

When you lose a child—no matter if it's an accident, illness, or some sudden, unthinkable tragedy—there's a part of you that doesn't come back. In Appalachia, that grief is often quiet, but it's everywhere. It sits in the pew at church next to you. It hangs in the air on your porch at night. It's in the way neighbors pause, wanting to say something but not knowing how.

Nationwide, 1 in every 12 children will lose a parent or sibling before turning eighteen[18]. Here in West Virginia—where the mountains seem to hold both our joys and our sorrows—nearly 19,000 children have lost a parent. That's about 5% of every child in the state[19].

The truth is, grief here often starts even earlier. In Appalachian Ohio, Kentucky, and West Virginia, the infant mortality rate is 7.4 per 1,000 live births—well above the national average of 6.1[20] [21]. Every one of those numbers is a name. A face. A family.

---

[18] National Alliance for Children's Grief. *Rural America and Childhood Bereavement.* https://n acg.org/ru ral-america

[19] Evermore. *State Fact Sheet: West Virginia.* https://ev ermore.org/w p-content/u ploads/2 022/1 1/W est-Virginia.pdf

[20] Appalachian Regional Commission. *Health Disparities in Appalachia: Child Health Domain.* https://w ww.arc.gov/w p-content/u ploads/2 021/0 2/H ealth_Disparities_in_Appalachia_Child_Health_Domain.pdf

[21] Penn State University. *Infant Mortality Rates Highlight Health Care Deficit in Appalachia.* https://w ww.psu.edu/n ew s/h ealth-and-human-development/s tory/a ppalachian-infant-death-rates-point-health-care-deficit

We're raised to be tough here, to "keep going." But that means a lot of grief in these mountains is disenfranchised—unspoken, unseen, and unacknowledged[22]. If you've ever buried a child, you know the truth: it doesn't matter how strong you are—this kind of loss changes you. And without a place to lay that grief down, you end up carrying it alone.

---

[22] Doka, Kenneth J. *Disenfranchised Grief*. Routledge,1989.

CHAPTER FOUR

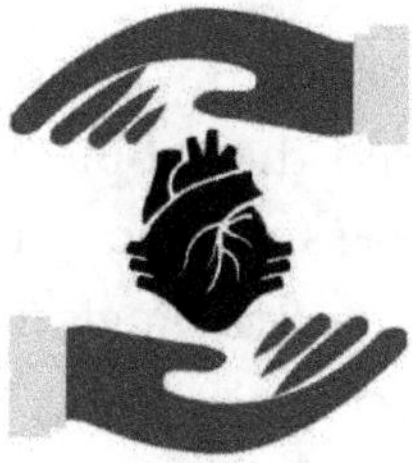

THE ANATOMY OF KINDNESS

"If you see someone without a smile, give them yours."

— Dolly Parton

In chaplaincy, we work under the premise of what's called *the living human document*—a concept at the very foundation of Clinical Pastoral Education, first given to us by its founder, Anton Boisen. Boisen believed that every person is a text to be read, their life written in the ink of joy, suffering, hope, and loss. Our task is to approach that text with the same reverence we'd bring to sacred scripture—listening for what is said, and for what is left unsaid.

Every time I encounter a family, I'm learning. I'm learning about them, about the human condition, and about myself. Each family—every individual—has been a teacher, offering something that has shaped me into a better advocate, a better husband, a better father, and, I hope, a better human being.

This was one of those cases where I walked away, reminded that there is something truly different about the people of Appalachia. At their core is a way of life rooted in kindness and hospitality. Even though I'm from Appalachian Ohio, my corner of the region is still very much part of the Northeast. The culture there feels more like New England than the South—everything is fast-paced, you don't make much eye contact when passing someone in the hallway or on the street, and conversations tend to be short and to the point. When I find myself in the southern Appalachian region, I have to remind myself to turn the Yankee off and blend into my surroundings—slowing down, softening my edges, and meeting people where they are.

I had an assignment on the opposite side of the state, in a different time zone. As chance would have it, they needed me to pack up my things and head east—there'd been an emergency, and one of the staff had to call off, so I grabbed my go bag and drove toward a small rural town with a hospital to match.

This was the kind of place that might see only one or two donors a month. Because of that, the hospital staff was eager to help in any way they could, offering the family every bit of support possible.

Several hours later, I checked into my hotel, took a quick shower, and opened my laptop. I saw I had about three hours until the organ recovery would take place. That meant I had a little time to breathe. I figured I could spare an hour, so I started flipping through TV channels and scrolling through TikTok, letting my mind idle for a moment before the next wave of work began.

As I was scrolling, I glanced up at the top right corner of my phone and froze. The organ recovery was in an hour—and the hospital was twenty minutes from my hotel.

What I hadn't accounted for when I looked at my laptop earlier was the time zone change. I had lost an hour without realizing it. Now, instead of easing into the evening, I was pressed for time, heading to a hospital I had never been to before, to meet a family I knew nothing about.

Not exactly the way you want to start a shift.

By some miracle, I made it on site and found my way to the Intensive Care Unit (ICU). I met with the Organ Recovery Coordinator (ORC) and learned two more small blessings: the OR was running on schedule, and we would be withdrawing in the Post-Anesthesia Care Unit (PACU) instead of the operating room. That gave me exactly what I needed to start my pre-OR conversation with the family.

I crossed the hall, gently knocked on the door, and asked permission to enter.

"Hi, my name is Brent," I began. "I'm the Family Services Coordinator who will be with you all this evening."

From across the room, someone called out, "You're not from around here, are you?"

I laughed. "Is my accent that noticeable?"

"That's correct," I added. "I'm from Ohio—just down here traveling to help out a bit."

One of the older women in the room grinned. "Oh, so they sent us a Yankee," she said with a chuckle.

I'm going to like these people, I thought to myself and said with a grin, "I'm afraid you're stuck with me.

If I understand correctly, you all wanted an honor walk?"

"Yes," the patient's brother, Eric, replied.

"And how many of you were planning on coming down to the PACU to be with Devin?"

"Well, they told us there can only be three people there," Eric said, "but we'd really like to have just a couple more."

It was a request I'd heard many times before. Sometimes we could make it happen; other times we couldn't. In the end, it always came down to the hospital and what they were willing to allow in that moment.

"I'll see what I can do," I said, and continued giving the family their instructions.

I went back to my clinical coordinator and asked if he'd call the OR to see if we could have a few more people come back. He made the call, and, to my surprise, they said they'd allow five. That was great news—I couldn't wait to walk back into that room and tell the family.

I returned to Devon's room to share the good news, and I barely got the first words out when Eric jumped in.

"We're going to need thirteen people in there."

Thirteen.

Okay, I thought to myself. How on earth am I going to negotiate thirteen? My clinical coordinator—who I'd met all of twenty minutes ago—is going to think I've completely lost my mind.

I walked back across the hall.

"Hey, Josh," I said.

"What's up, man?" he replied, turning toward me. Then he caught the look on my face. "What happened?"

"So… how big is the PACU?" I asked.

Josh narrowed his eyes. "Why?"

"Thirteen," I said flatly. "I need thirteen people to fit in that room."

He shook his head. "Bro, I am not calling the OR back. They're going to kill me."

"I can call them," I offered.

"No, man, I'll call—but you're going to owe me."

He dialed. No answer. And time was running short. The honor walk was moments away, people already lining the halls. Dozens of Devon's family and friends kept pouring onto the unit—hugging, crying, telling stories. I'd never seen a community rally around someone the way they did for him that night. It was inspiring to hear all the lives he'd touched.

But in the back of my mind, I was still turning over the same problem—how to get thirteen people into the PACU without ending up in trouble with the hospital.

So, I did what any Family Services Coordinator would do—I decided to wing it.

The honor walk began, and we started moving down the hallway. The family followed... but so did everyone else. All the extended family. Friends. Neighbors. By the time I looked back, there were thirty people in all.

I drifted toward the back, doing a little crowd control, when I met Devon's cousin Bill.

"Man, this is pretty amazing," Bill said, eyes scanning the hallway lined with nurses, doctors, and staff standing in silence.

"It really is," I agreed.

"So, this is what you get to do every day?" he asked.

"Yeah," I said, "I have the honor of doing this and walking with families like yours every day."

"How do you get into work like this?" he asked.

"Well, I was a hospital chaplain before this," I explained. "It was kind of a natural progression for me."

"Were you a chaplain here?"

"No," I smiled. "Back home in Ohio."

"Ohio! How did you end up here?" Bill asked, eyebrows raised.

"Well," I said, "I get to travel around the country doing this. I used to manage a team of people who do this work, but then my wife got sick. I took some time off to be with her and stepped away from my organization back home. Once she got her clean bill of health, I decided I wanted to start traveling around the country doing this."

Bill grabbed his wife's hand and said, "Honey, listen to this. Tell her what you do for a living—how you get to travel all over the country doing this."

"Yeah," I said. "It's pretty amazing. I never in a million years thought I'd be traveling across the country doing this kind of work."

"His wife got sick, and now that she's better, he's traveling," Bill added.

"What happened?" his wife, Cindy, asked.

"She was diagnosed with breast cancer," I answered, keeping it short. I didn't want to pull their focus away from why we were all really there—their cousin. This wasn't the time to weigh the air down with my story.

"Oh my," Cindy said softly. "But she's all better now?"

"Yeah," I replied. "She's got a clean bill of health."

Cindy smiled, her voice carrying that mix of relief and gentle insistence only a wife can give. "Well, you make sure you go back to Ohio and spoil her when you're finished here."

I laughed, the heaviness of the conversation lifting for just a second. "Absolutely," I said.

As we approached the elevator doors, I turned back and realized we'd picked up more than just the immediate family. A whole crowd had formed behind us—cousins, aunts, uncles, friends. Way more than the thirteen I had been planning to squeeze in. The honor walk had taken on a life of its own, and in that moment, it felt less like logistics and more like a procession.

We still had to go down one floor to reach the operating suite. It was clear it would take multiple elevators to make this happen, so one by one, family, friends, and neighbors piled in and descended the two floors. My clinical team, escorting Devon's bed, waited for everyone to arrive before we began the short walk to the OR doors.

This was the place where I customarily paused and gave families space for their final goodbyes before the donor was taken back for preparation. Afterward, I would escort the family to the room where the extubation would take place.

I always use this moment to remind families that we are crossing into a sacred space. I tell them that I am a guest—there to assist, more a silent observer than a participant—stepping in only when needed or when invited. I encourage them to take the time to do what they need: play music, pray, speak the words that have gone unsaid.

Devon was escorted back to the OR by the clinical team while the rest of us waited outside. After a few moments, we were given the all-clear to come in. The original thirteen went back, but Bill and Cindy, along with another nine or ten people, stayed behind.

"You're not going back?" I asked Bill.

"I'd like to," Bill said, "but it's more important that those other folks go."

I had already been back to the PACU to help with preparations, and I knew it was completely empty. There was room back there for fifty—maybe seventy-five—people, so I did something I don't normally do.

"Bill," I said, lowering my voice with a small grin, "I was never one for math growing up, and I'm not sure how many people have already gone back. I'm going to head back there—and I think you folks should follow me."

"Really?" Bill asked, his eyebrows lifting.

"Yes," I said simply.

The group followed me back into the room where Devon lay. By then, per the family's wishes, he had already been extubated. Around his bed sat a circle of older relatives and lifelong friends, their chairs pulled close, hands resting on the rails or folded in their laps. Behind them stood another ring—Devon's closest friends, hovering just beyond the bedside, leaning in with quiet reverence. Further back, forming a third circle, were the extended family and neighbors. That's where I stood, at the edge, with Bill and Cindy beside me.

It was there, in that outer circle, that Bill began to ask me questions about the donation process.

"So what happens now?" Bill asked quietly.

"We wait," I replied. "We allow Devon to pass naturally, just as he would in the ICU if he weren't a donor."

I paused, then continued, "Once he passes, I'll escort you all out, andwe'll return to the room to gather your belongings. After that, the organ recovery will begin. Devon is donating his kidneys and his liver—he'll be saving two lives today, provided he passes within sixty minutes."

"Why sixty minutes?" Cindy asked.

"It has to do with blood flow and oxygen reaching the organs," I explained gently. "After a certain point, the organs aren't getting enough to remain healthy. Beyond that window, they're no longer viable for transplant."

I do my best to balance pastoral care with clinical expertise when working with families. Over the years, through chaplaincy and now in donation work, I've learned that clear, clinical explanations often serve families best. When they understand the process, step by step, it brings a measure of peace to the chaos. The mystery doesn't feel so threatening when it's explained plainly.

Language matters. If I speak in medical jargon, they may nod politely but carry away confusion. But if I take the time to translate—oxygen instead of O_2 saturation, time limits instead of ischemia—they can truly grasp what's happening. And when they understand, they can make sense of their loved one's gift.

It's always easy for us to slip into medical jargon. We speak it daily with our colleagues and hospital partners—it becomes second nature. But as donation advocates, entrusted with the honor of walking alongside donor families, we must resist that instinct. Our responsibility is to meet families where they are, to speak in words they can hold onto, and to make sure they have every piece of information they need and every answer they ask for.

"What do those numbers mean on the screen over there?" Cindy asked, pointing toward the monitor.

I stepped a little closer so she could see where I was looking. "These numbers are telling us about Devon's heart rate, his oxygen level, and his blood pressure," I explained. "They're the vital signs the team follows. Right now, we're watching for changes that will let us know when his body is beginning to let go."

I kept my tone gentle, careful not to overwhelm with detail, but steady enough to honor her question. Families notice everything in those moments—the lights, the alarms, the screens. A simple explanation can turn something intimidating into something they can hold in their hands and understand.

"Thank you, Brent," Cindy said softly.

"You're welcome," I replied. "This is what I'm here for."

She shook her head slightly, her eyes still on the monitor. "I don't know how you do this every day."

I gave a small smile. "Some days, I don't either," I admitted. "But every family deserves someone to walk with them through this. That's what keeps me showing up."

Some glad morning, when this life is over…

The sound filled the room, and before long others joined in. One after another, voices lifted until the hymn swelled around Devon's bed:

I'll fly away, oh glory,

I'll fly away;

When I die, hallelujah by and by,

I'll fly away.

The room, heavy with silence just moments before, became a sanctuary of song. Grief and hope braided together in the voices of family and friends, carrying Devon on the only procession that mattered.

By the final verse, it wasn't just the family singing. We were all singing—doctors, nurses, family, friends, and organ procurement staff—our voices joining together in that small, crowded PACU room. In that moment, there were no roles or titles, no dividing lines between professional and personal. We stood together as witnesses, bound by the sacred weight of farewell, recognizing the holiness of what was unfolding before us.

A few moments later, Devon's stats began to show that his body was letting go. I gently encouraged the family to start saying their goodbyes. One by one, they stepped forward—kissing him, whispering prayers, laying a hand on his arm, speaking final words of love.

It was fitting, almost beyond words. As if the Spirit itself had chosen the time. Devon's family and friends had just sent him off with his favorite hymn, and now, surrounded by love and song, he slipped toward the life beyond.

It is moments like these that remind me of the sacredness of the work we do. In donation, we often find ourselves standing in the thin space between what is natural and what is holy. Death and life, sorrow and hope, humanity and divinity—all of it converges in these rooms. And in bearing witness, I am reminded, again and again, that this work is not only clinical, but sacred.

Devon's story did not end with his final breath. His story lives on in the two recipients who rose from their own hospital beds with the gift of life beating within them. For his family, that hymn and that sacred farewell will always be their memory of him. For the recipients, his legacy is written into every tomorrow they now have. And for me, it is another reminder that a single "yes" can echo far beyond the walls of a hospital room.

CHAPTER FIVE

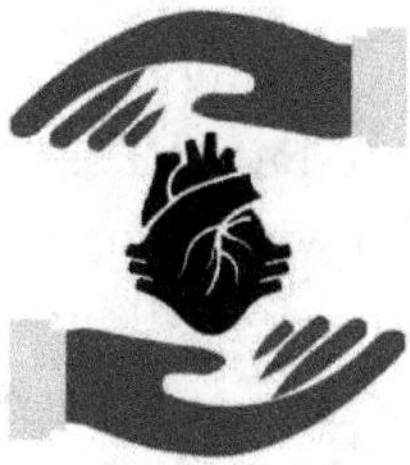

THE ANATOMY OF REDEMPTION

"Every saint has a past, and every sinner has a future."

— *Oscar Wilde*

In June of 2020, my brother Eric walked to McDonald's for what should have been an ordinary day. Somewhere along that walk, his body betrayed him. A massive seizure overtook him on the street.

Eric was known in the community, but not for anything that would earn him mercy in that moment. He carried the label of "addict," and so when the police found him convulsing, they assumed the worst. To them, he wasn't a man in crisis — he was overdosing, combative, a problem to be subdued. By the time the paramedics arrived, my brother had taken a beating on top of the storm already raging inside his brain. It wasn't until then that someone recognized what was actually happening: this wasn't drugs, this was a seizure. This was the first sign of the brain cancer that would change his life, and ours, forever.

That week in the hospital, we finally had a name for what had taken my brother down in the street: a Grade III astrocytoma. The doctors didn't sugarcoat his prognosis. Even with surgery, he was given the estimate of one to two years. Grim words to swallow for anyone, but especially for Eric. Layered on top of this was another reality he couldn't escape — the weight of his addiction had left him with legal troubles, and a prison sentence of two years was already waiting for him just months away. Faced with that, Eric made a decision that was his alone to make. He chose not to undergo surgery. He would walk into the days ahead without illusions, determined to live them fully, even with the shadow of prison looming.

Eric and I corresponded through email nearly every day, and we spoke on the phone once a week. Those conversations became a lifeline between us, a way to hold on to something normal in the midst of everything that wasn't. In those exchanges, I began to learn the truth of what his life inside really looked like. The prison was often running out of his medication. Appointments that had been scheduled were missed or ignored. The medical care he received was, at best, inadequate. For a man carrying a terminal brain cancer diagnosis, it was less than ideal — it was cruel.

During the first year of his incarceration, I placed more than one hundred calls to the warden's office, each one an attempt to advocate for my brother's care. Not a single call was ever returned. Every time, I spoke with the warden's assistant, and every time, she assured me she would pass along the message for him to call me back. He never did. With each unanswered attempt, I was reminded again of how powerless we were against a system that had already decided what Eric was worth.

In April of the following year, life gave me a brief reprieve from hospitals, phone calls, and worry, or so I thought. My daughter had just turned sixteen, and we were celebrating in style. We had rented out the local movie theater for the afternoon and planned a 1950s-themed party, complete with the musical *Hairspray* on the big screen. Everyone was dressed in their best period outfits — poodle skirts, saddle shoes, and letterman jackets — laughter and anticipation filling the air.

We caravanned in two separate vehicles, a car full of teenagers in tow. Somewhere along the way, my phone rang. It was my brother's girlfriend. With the car packed to the brim, I let it roll over to voicemail. Moments later, it rang again. This time, I answered.

Before I could even say hello, I heard her voice: *"Eric had a massive seizure."*

"Oh my God—when and where is he?" I asked, gripping the steering wheel tighter.

"I don't know," she said. *"I just got a call from his bunkie."*

"Do we know if he's okay?" I pressed.

"All he was able to tell me before the call cut out was that Eric had a massive seizure. It took them twenty minutes to get to him, and he still wasn't awake when they arrived."

Silence filled the car for a beat, the teenagers in the backseat laughing and oblivious to the storm breaking on the other end of the line.

"Shit. Okay. I'll call you back," I said, already bracing myself for what would come next.

Working in donation, you come to understand pretty quickly what the lack of oxygen does to the brain. It's not just medical knowledge; it's lived knowledge, carried from hospital rooms and ICU bedsides. I knew what twenty minutes without response could mean. I knew what that kind of seizure could leave behind. As much as I wanted to hold on to hope in that moment, a part of me already understood the weight of what we were facing.

We arrived at the theater, the kids fighting over who got to sit next to who — my wife still in the dark about what was happening, and me doing my best to keep a sense of normalcy so as not to ruin the day. The lights dimmed, the screen flickered to life, and the kids, buzzing in their 1950s outfits, were swept up in the moment. They sang along with that opening line — "Good morning, Baltimore" — their enthusiasm rising above the music. I finally had my chance to step away, the weight of knowing what I was about to walk into pressing hard against my chest. I then began making the calls I knew I had to make.

The first call I made was to my mom. My dad had passed away the year before, and as I dialed her number, I couldn't help but feel the sting of déjà vu — this was all too reminiscent of the call I had once made to my brother in prison. Somehow, because I am the one who works around death, these calls always fall to me. It's a burden I rarely want, but one I seem to carry again and again.

"Mom, Eric's had a seizure. He was down for twenty minutes or so, and I'm not sure where they've taken him. I'm going to try and get ahold of the prison. I'll call you back."

I got all of this out in a single breath, trying to steady my tone so it wouldn't betray the panic rising in me. On the other end of the line, I could hear my mother's sobs breaking through, her tears filling the silence I couldn't hold for her. I ended the call and immediately started dialing the prison. No answer. I called again. Still nothing... again and again — each ring only deepening the silence.

I started frantically googling numbers for the prison, calling any number that might connect me to someone who knew what was happening. I tried the chaplain's office — nothing. The main switchboard — nothing. Finally, buried in a corner of the website, I found a number listed for medical professionals needing to reach the nurse on duty.

I dialed the number. *Ring. Ring.* The sound was tinny, old-fashioned, like the phones that used to hang on the wall with rotary dials. It rang and rang, but no one ever picked up. I hung up and tried the main switchboard one last time. This time, finally, someone answered.

"Department of Corrections, this is [name]."

I gave my name, explained who I was, and why I was calling. His reply was flat, almost rehearsed: *"Sorry, there's no one in medical today. You'll have to call back Monday."*

The waiting was eternal.

This wasn't a case, or a shift, or a file number. This was my brother.

And I felt helpless. There was nothing we could do except wait, and every hour stretched like it wanted to break me.

On Monday, I called again, hoping maybe this time someone would answer with news that wasn't another wall. No luck. Just silence.

I didn't know what else I could do, so I started calling some of my friends in law enforcement, explaining the situation—not as a professional, but as a brother. I asked if they knew anyone, anyone at all, who could help me break through the barricade of unanswered phones and closed doors.

They gave me the number for the state department of corrections' medical director. I called. No answer. Called again. Nothing.

We kept running into dead ends. Every call felt like pushing on a locked door. Every silence felt heavier than the one before.

And when it's your own family, silence is not neutral. Silence is cruelty. It's the sound of hope eroding in real time.

I finally tracked down a number for a state senate oversight group that monitored the department of corrections. I don't even remember how I found it—probably some corner of a government website I'd stared at for too long—but I dialed, not knowing what to expect.

A staffer answered.

I told him everything. Calmly. Clearly. Like I'd practiced. Like it wasn't my brother we were talking about.

I explained how no one was giving us information. How every number we'd tried had gone nowhere. How my family was sitting in a fog of silence while time just kept stretching. I wasn't asking for favors. I was asking for decency. For answers.

He listened.

Then he said something that gave me the first flicker of hope I'd felt in days.

"You're not going to believe this," he said, "but we're actually walking into a meeting about healthcare issues in the Department of Corrections—this morning. I'll make sure this gets raised."

I hung up the phone and didn't move for hours.

I sat by that phone like it was a lifeline. I must have checked the volume a dozen times, kept it in my hand like it might vanish if I let go. But the hours passed, and the silence returned.

Nothing came that day.

Then—Tuesday morning—my phone rang. Restricted number.

I knew it had to be someone.

I answered. "Hello?"

A man's voice on the other end, sharp but not unkind.

"This is Dr. [Name], Director of Medical Services for the State Department of Corrections. You apparently have some friends in high places—your brother's name landed on my desk this morning with a note that said: 'Call this guy.' So here I am."

When it's your own family, you feel the weight of every unanswered call like a punch. You hear every "we'll call you back" as a hollow promise. You realize what it feels like to be on the outside of the system looking in—and it is terrifying.

Thankfully, my brother got the help he needed. I was able to advocate, to press, to find the names and numbers buried beneath layers of bureaucracy. But that experience didn't leave me unchanged.

If anything, it sharpened me.

It taught me that behind every correctional facility, every security checkpoint, every inmate number—there is a family. A sister. A mother. A brother pacing the floor, clutching their phone like it's a lifeline.

And it taught me something else: That dignity doesn't come with qualifications.

It belongs to everyone.

That moment became a turning point in my work. I started seeing the people others look past. I found myself at bedside meetings with prison wardens and state correctional medical staff, facilitating donation conversations in the unlikeliest of places—with families who never imagined they'd be asked to make a decision so sacred under circumstances so complex.

But I was ready. Because I'd lived it.

And I carried that memory with me—not as a wound, but as a reminder. A reminder to never let paperwork overshadow personhood. To never let a uniform or a sentence or a record strip away the fundamental truth that every life carries value. Every loss carries grief. Every yes carries weight.

Little did I know what my experience would prepare me for.

Several months later I was called to the hospital for an approach. The patient was a prisoner who had been assaulted by another inmate. He had been declared brain dead, and his family was gathered at the bedside.

When I arrived, I huddled with the nurse before meeting the attending. "Just so you know, this guy is one of the worst," she began, launching into what he was in prison for.

I stopped her gently. "There's no need to tell me. I'm not here to judge his past—I'm here to offer his family a little bit of hope."

"Well, you need to know what he did. And so do the recipients. They have a right to know," she insisted.

"I disagree," I said. "He served his time, and ultimately, he died for whatever he did. Something inside him told him to say 'yes' to donation—maybe he was trying to right his wrongs. Either way, I don't need to know what he did. My role is to support his family and walk with them through this process."

I met with the attending and explained why I was there. He told me that before I could move forward, I would need to call and speak with the warden.

I was confused. The patient had died. I assumed the state would no longer have any say in what happened. I was wrong.

Unfortunately, the warden made it clear, death did not change anything in his eyes. The patient was still a ward of the state, still a prisoner, and the warden was going to make sure everyone knew it.

"I understand," I said, though inside I didn't. "I'm going to go call Warden Jones now and talk to him."

I went to the room to see the patient. The family had not yet arrived from out of state, so I had some time to make the necessary calls. Whenever possible, I like to see the patient—the donor—before I meet with the family. It's a grounding practice for me, a reminder that this is a human being, and that they deserve dignity and respect.

When I entered the room, I was stunned. The patient—his name was Brian—was still handcuffed to the bed. A prison guard stood stationed just outside the door.

I introduced myself to the guard, explaining that I would be speaking with the family and that Brian was a registered donor. Then I asked the question that was burning inside me: *Why is he still handcuffed? He's dead.*

The guard didn't flinch. "Well, he's a prisoner, and we have to make sure he doesn't escape."

"Did they let you know that Brian has been declared brain dead?" I asked.

"Yes, I know Offender Smith is dead," he replied flatly. "But he is to remain handcuffed until I am told otherwise."

He was cold and matter-of-fact. I imagine it comes from the things he witnesses every day, a kind of armor built from routine and necessity. But still—Brian wasn't going anywhere. He was dead. The cuffs didn't make sense to me.

"Well, I think I need to speak to Warden Jones now and see how we're going to proceed," I said. I left the room and found a small, empty conference room. As I sat down, I felt almost a flashback—memories of trying to reach this same man when my brother was having all of his issues. But this time was different: I had his cell phone number. It would be harder for him to avoid me.

The phone rang. He answered. "Warden Jones." His voice carried a trace of a Southern drawl. He definitely wasn't from around here.

"Hi, Warden Jones," I said. "My name is Brent. I work with the organ procurement organization, and I'm calling about Mr. Smith, who is a registered donor—"

He cut me off. "Offender Smith is still a ward of the state, and I'll be making the decision to donate or not once I speak with Offender Smith's family."

"I totally understand, sir. Mr. Smith's family—"

"Offender Smith," he interrupted again, his correction sharp.

"Yes sir—Brian Smith—who was declared brain dead this afternoon, is a registered organ donor. Once his family arrives, I would like to speak with them regarding Brian's registry status and what that means moving forward."

There was silence on the other end of the line. Finally, he said, "I spoke to our legal team. If they are fine with donation, you can proceed with *Offender Smith's* donation."

The call ended abruptly.

My heart was pounding, and I noticed my palms were damp with sweat. I had finally come face-to-face—if only by phone—with the man who had dodged me so many times when I was advocating for my brother's health care during his incarceration.

This isn't meant as an indictment of the correctional system. Rather, it's an inside look at a reality most people will never witness—how the unique life experiences we carry as donation advocates shape the way we show up for others each time we step foot into a hospital.

Brian's sisters arrived not long after. I was introduced to two women, both in their thirties—Jennifer and Erica. They looked exhausted, worn down, defeated.

"Hi, my name is Brent. I'm part of the end-of-life care team—"

Before I could finish, Erica burst into tears. Jennifer, holding herself together just enough to speak, said, "You'll have to excuse us. We're a bit emotional. We've been trying to get information on Brian for days, and then we finally get a call from the hospital—and they tell us he's dead. Why didn't they call us sooner? We could have come and been with him."

This could have been me. I could have been sitting in their place, having the same conversation with a colleague. My heart broke for them.

"I know there's nothing I can say that will take away the pain," I told them. "And I can't begin to imagine what you are going through. I know you've just driven a couple of hours to get here, and you haven't even had time to simply be with Brian. What we need to talk about can wait. Take this time together as a family, and I'll come back later."

I stepped out and gave them their space. A nurse came up to me and asked what the sisters had decided. I explained that we hadn't talked yet—that I wanted to give them time with their brother—and that they were still very upset.

She said she would order some coffee and snacks for them. I asked if she might also call the chaplain.

"Thank you for taking care of the family," I told her. She gave a small nod and walked away.

After about thirty minutes, I returned to the room and sat with Jennifer and Erica. Gently, I shared with them that Brian was a registered organ donor. I explained the life-saving impact of that decision—how, even in death, he now had the ability to help many others through the gift of donation.

They both began to cry, and I moved my chair in closer.

"I don't know what Brian did to end up in prison," I said softly. "But what I do know is this—despite all of that, he made the choice to help others. To me, that is redemption. And it's something you, as his family, can be proud of."

The case of Brian's donation underscores a reality few outside of our field ever encounter. In the United States, the policies around organ donation for incarcerated individuals are inconsistent at best. Only about 40 percent of correctional systems even have clear donation guidelines.[23] Among those, fewer than half allow registration for posthumous donation, and many restrict living donations to immediate family members only.[24] Even the Federal Bureau of Prisons prohibits its inmates from registering as posthumous donors.[25] This patchwork of rules often leaves families, advocates, and even care teams navigating murky territory when time and clarity are most needed.

And yet, within those same prison walls, the willingness is there. Studies show that nearly three-quarters of inmates have a positive attitude toward organ donation, sixty percent would consent to donate a deceased family member's organs, and more than eighty percent expressed trust in the medical and transplant communities.[26] For people who are often treated only as numbers or case files, that trust and willingness speak volumes. It reminds us that dignity, compassion, and a desire to help others are not extinguished by incarceration.

---

[23] "Organ Donation Policies Among U.S. Carceral Systems," *National Library of Medicine*, 2023, https://p mc.ncbi.nlm.nih.gov/a rticles/P MC9996393.

[24] Scott Halpern et al., "U.S. Prison Policies on Organ Donation for Individuals Who Are Incarcerated," *JAMA Network Open* 6, no. 2 (2023, https://j amanetwork.com/j ournals/j amanetworkopen/f ullarticle/2 802129.

[25] Ibid.

[26] "Attitudes of Inmates Toward Organ Donation," *ResearchGate*, 2025, https://w ww.researchgate.net/p ublication/3 69091820_US_Prison_Policies_on_Organ_Donation_for_Individuals_Who_Are_Incarcerated.

The potential impact is staggering. One ethical analysis estimated that if just one percent of the roughly 2.2 million people incarcerated in the U.S. donated, it could yield around 21,000 kidneys.[27] That is not a statistic to be dismissed lightly. It represents thousands of lives restored, families kept whole, and communities healed. But the barriers—legal, ethical, and cultural—continue to prevent this potential from being realized. Concerns around coercion, informed consent, and systemic inequities must be weighed carefully, but they should not blind us to the humanity and agency of those behind prison walls.

Brian's story is a reminder of that humanity. To this day I don't know why Brian was in prison. But regardless of the why, it did not erase his capacity to choose yes for donation. Perhaps this was his story of redemption. Maybe he was trying to right his wrongs and show his sisters and those who loved him that he cared about others.

Brian's story, my brothers story, and the countless other stories just like theirs is a reminder for us as donation advocates that our role is more than just advocating for donation; it is a call to continue showing up—with dignity, with respect, and with a commitment to honoring every *yes*, no matter where it comes from.

---

[27] "Organ Donation Policies Among U.S. Carceral Systems," *National Library of Medicine*, 2023, https://p mc.ncbi.nlm.nih.gov/a rticles/P MC9996393.

CHAPTER SIX

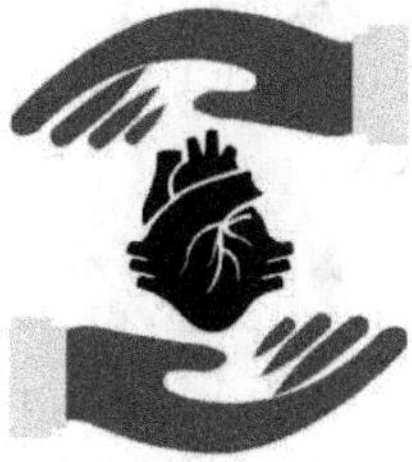

THE ANATOMY OF A NO

"Pain insists upon being attended to. God whispers to us in our pleasures, speaks in our conscience, but shouts in our pains: it is his megaphone to rouse a deaf world."

-C.S.Lewis (*The Problem of Pain*)

The Anatomy of a No may sound like a strange chapter to find in a book called *The Anatomy of a Yes*. But despite my best efforts and advocacy, I do not always hear "yes" from families. To pretend otherwise would be dishonest. I would be doing you, the reader, a disservice if I didn't invite you into one of those rooms — a room where donation was declined, and where my role was not to secure an outcome, but simply to bear witness.

This next story is one that remains seared into my memory. It flashes back into my mind every time I step into a pediatric ICU. It is the story of Emily — or as her parents called her, simply, Em.

I was across the hospital on the adult side when the call came in for me to head over to the pediatric hospital. An eight-year-old girl had just been admitted that morning, and now her family was preparing to withdraw care. So, I made my way over.

I dread these approaches. They are never easy. Nothing about them feels natural. It is unnatural to see a child who has died. Unnatural to watch parents carry that grief so heavily. And yet, this is part of the work — walking into rooms that were never meant to exist.

But these rooms do exist. And when they do, we are called to walk into them — balancing the tightrope of advocacy and empathy, presence and purpose.

So I went, determined to give my best — to honor the family grieving before me and the patients waiting on the transplant list. When I arrived on the unit, I huddled with a group of residents and the bedside nurse. My first question was simple: *What happened?*

"Unwitnessed asthma attack," one of the residents answered. "She went to the bathroom and was gone for a few minutes, so the teacher sent another student to check. That's when she was found. Help was called right away, but by the time they reached her, it was too late."

Two thoughts immediately crossed my mind. First, this poor child likely had no idea what was happening when she walked into that bathroom. And second, the trauma is now carried by the student who found her.

Two children forever marked — one whose life was cut short, and another whose childhood was shattered in an instant.

So here we were, twenty-four hours post admission. The care team had just completed the second round of brain death testing, and the parents had just been given the devastating news: their daughter was gone.

You could feel the sorrow pouring into the hallway, as if the grief itself had substance. It was thick, heavy, filling every corner of the ICU. The sound of their sobbing cut through the background of monitors and conversations, rising above the sound of the machines. This sound was the unmistakable cry of parents whose world had just been shattered.

Now, the sacred duty of sharing with these parents the opportunity for their daughter to live on through organ donation rested on my shoulders. I have heard countless donor parents speak of the healing that donation brought them, and I carry those stories with me into every approach.

But knowing that truth does not make these conversations any easier. You place yourself in their shoes, and you recognize that you are stepping in only thirty minutes after their world has been forever changed. The weight of that timing is immense. It demands that I set aside everything else and do my best to honor both the enormity of their loss and the possibility of legacy that donation represents.

I knocked gently on the door before entering. The room was crowded, every space already claimed by sorrow and those trying to hold it together.

The attending stood at Emily's bedside, steady and solemn. Across from him, the social worker and nurse practitioner lingered, their presence a quiet anchor. On the floor sat her mother and father, broken open by grief, each flanked by a child life specialist who was doing everything possible to hold them upright in the storm.

They were all there, all silent, and all eyes on me. The air was thick with expectation, the kind of silence that makes every second feel heavier.

Before I could speak, the attending broke it. "This is Brent," he said gently. "He's from the organ procurement organization, and he will be talking with you about the possibility of Emily being a donor."

In that moment, I felt a rush of gratitude. Gratitude that he had broken the silence, and gratitude that he trusted me enough to carry this most delicate conversation with her parents.

"Mr. and Mrs. Adams," I began softly, "I am so terribly sorry to be meeting you under these circumstances. I can't even begin to imagine what you are going through."

"Thank you," Mr. Adams said quietly.

"As Dr. Jones mentioned, I am part of the organ procurement organization, and I'm here to share some information with you."

At that, Mrs. Adams let out an audible cry, the sound tearing through the room in a way that words never could.

"We've been talking about it," Mr. Adams said. "Dr. Jones let us know you would be coming in. So we have some questions we'd like to ask before we make a decision, if that's okay."

"Absolutely," I replied. "Do you mind if I sit with you?"

"Please," he said.

So I lowered myself onto the floor beside them, meeting them at eye level in their grief. "What questions do you have?" I asked gently.

"What organs would you harvest?" Mr. Adams asked.

"On every potential donor we evaluate the eight life-saving gifts," I explained softly, "the heart, liver, lungs, pancreas, kidneys, and intestines."

Mr. Adams swallowed hard, his eyes wet. "I don't know, Carol," he said to his wife, voice breaking. "I don't know that I can do this."

She reached for his hand. "John, if we can save another family from going through this, we should."

"I just don't like the idea of them… cutting her apart," he whispered.

Normally, this is where I would step in — to reassure them, to explain the care and dignity with which recovery surgeons treat every donor. But now was not the time. They weren't asking for education yet. They were wrestling, right there on the floor, with a decision no parent ever wants to make. And in that moment, my role was not to interrupt, but to bear witness to the sacred and to answer only when asked.

Mr. Adams turned toward me, his voice trembling. "How… how do they do the surgery?"

I nodded gently, placing a hand on my own chest to demonstrate. "It's done through a single midline incision," I explained softly, tracing from the bottom of my breastbone to the top of my belly button. "The recovery surgeons are extremely respectful. They treat every donor with dignityand respect — we view our donors as heroes, and they are cared for with the deepest respect."

"Carol, it's not right. I don't think I can do this," Mr. Adams said as he stood up abruptly and began pacing the room.

I rose with him, keeping my voice gentle. "Mr. Adams, I want you to know — there is no pressure. There is no right or wrong answer here. I'm here to walk with you and support you, no matter what you decide."

"John," Carol said softly, "let's ask our other questions, so we at least know."

She turned toward me. "How long will this process take if we decide to go through with it?"

"Donation is a process," I explained gently. "We would begin with a series of blood draws and a review of Emily's medical records. Then we would work to match her gifts with the recipients who need them most. You would be able to remain present with her the entire time. She would stay in this same room until it is time for the recovery."

"Would this happen today?" Mrs. Adams asked, her voice fragile.

"It would not," I replied. "We would ask that you keep the ventilator on while we work through the process. Most likely, she would go to the operating room for recovery tomorrow or the following day."

She suddenly burst into tears. "I don't think I can keep seeing her like this. She's gone, and I know she's gone. Keeping her on these machines feels cruel — cruel to her and hell for us."

I leaned in gently, lowering my voice. "I'm so sorry. I know this is so much information, and I know that donation is an enormous ask — especially in the middle of unimaginable grief. The ventilator would need to remain on to ensure her organs stay healthy enough for transplantation."

"I want to assure you that we do everything we can to move as quickly as possible — both to honor your *yes* and to ensure that we help as many people as possible," I said, "but I also want to make sure I answer every question you have, and that you have the space and time you need to talk before making a decision. What other questions can I answer for you?"

Mr. Adams shook his head gently. "I think that's all for now. Can we please have some time to talk it over?"

"You most certainly can," I replied. "I'll be at the nurses' station whenever you're ready to reconvene."

I was only three months off orientation when I was assigned this case. Brand new to the role, still finding my footing, and suddenly standing in the middle of one of the hardest conversations of my career. This was one of my first pediatric approaches, and it seared itself into my memory.

Looking back now, with years of experience behind me, I can see so many places where I might have pivoted differently — where I could have created more space, slowed the pace, and allowed the family more room to breathe before asking them to decide. At the time, I was doing my best with the tools I had, but grief is a teacher, and this family taught me lessons that have shaped every approach since.

I tend to be very clinical in my approaches. By that, I don't mean I overwhelm families with medical jargon, but rather that I am concise and matter-of-fact. There is a reason for this.

Early in my career as a trauma chaplain, I learned that packaging devastating news in flowery language can cloud the truth. Euphemisms like *"passed away"* or *"no longer with us"* may soften the words for the speaker, but they can confuse families about the seriousness of the prognosis — sometimes even planting seeds of false hope.

So, I choose clarity. Instead of saying, *"your loved one has passed,"* I name it for what it is: *"your loved one has died."* It feels stark, but it is honest. And in moments where everything is already spinning, honesty is the first mercy we can offer.

We have to remember, after all, that we are agents of mercy in these situations. We are called to stand in the tension between life and death — death on the donor side and life on the recipient side. And in that sacred space, our task is not only to advocate for the gift of life, but to extend mercy to the families before us. Mercy in how we speak, mercy in how we listen, and mercy in how we honor their decisions, whatever they may be.

Earlier in the book, I spoke about the idea of the living human document—the principle that we learn more through our direct encounters with families than we ever could in a classroom. This concept comes from Anton Boisen, who is considered the founder of Clinical Pastoral Education (CPE). In the early days of CPE, Boisen emphasized that "reading 'the living human documents'" was a vital complement to seminary classroom work, asserting that the study of human experience must augment theological training.[28] His insight has shaped generations of chaplains by grounding our pastoral formation in real, lived stories rather than classroom instruction and theory alone. And it has not only shaped me into the donation advocate that I am today, but also influenced every donation advocate I have had the privilege of training.

As I sat at the nurses' station waiting to be called back into the room, I found myself doing what I used to do after every chaplain's visit. I replayed the conversation in my mind, word for word, over and over again, studying how I entered their sacred space. Did I show empathy at

---

[28] Anton T. Boisen, *The Biography of Anton Theophilus Boisen*, Association for Clinical Pastoral Education, Inc.

the right moments? Where did I listen well, and where might I have rushed the conversation along because I was uncomfortable? What did I do right, and where were the opportunities for growth?

The waiting stretched on, each minute feeling like an eternity. I truly didn't know which way the parents were leaning. Would they say yes, and be willing to walk this journey of donation? Or would the reality of keeping Emily on the ventilator become the barrier that stopped them from moving forward? Their grief was raw, their questions fragile. All I could do was hope that I had offered enough compassion to meet them in their pain, while still holding space for the recipients who depended on me to advocate on their behalf.

Bethany, Emily's nurse, walked over quietly. She placed her hand on my shoulder, and said, "They're ready for you, Brent."

I knocked gently on the door. "Is it okay if I come in?" I asked.

"Please," Mrs. Adams said. Then, almost immediately, she broke into tears. "I'm so sorry…"

"Brent, we just can't do this," Mr. Adams said, stepping in, his voice breaking as tears filled his eyes. "We just can't keep her like this. And we feel guilty, because we know we have the ability to make other parents not have to go through this. But… we're being selfish."

I shook my head gently. "Mr. Adams, you are not being selfish. You know your limits, and this decision is yours alone. The fact that you were even willing to talk with me in this moment speaks volumes about the kind and caring people you are. I am so very sorry for your loss. I only wish there were something I could do or say to take away even a part of the pain you're experiencing."

He nodded, tears still streaming. "Brent, you've been very kind, and we appreciate that."

With that, I exited the room and called my team to let them know. I offered Bethany a few simple instructions and then left the hospital. In the parking deck, I sat for a long while, listening to music and replaying the conversation in my mind, over and over again.

In the years since that night, I have had many families say no. Some of them have followed up with me weeks, even months later, to tell me that they wished they had the chance to revisit the decision. More than once I've heard, *"If we could go back, we would have said yes."*

Those conversations have never left me. They make me wonder: could I have done or said something differently in that moment to help them see the possibility of donation? Or were they simply not ready, and the no was the only answer they could give at the time?

Over time, what I have come to understand is that a "no" is not the end of the story. I've learned that grief has a way of changing with time, and families often revisit the decisions they made in the rawest hours of loss. Research confirms what I have seen firsthand: nearly sixteen percent of families who initially declined donation later expressed regret, wishing they could go back and make a different choice.[29] By contrast, families who consented to donation almost never reported regret. This does not

---

[29]Laura Jane Morrison, et al. "Family Experiences and Regret Following Organ Donation Decisions: A Retrospective Study." *Australian Critical Care*, 2025. https://www.sciencedirect.com/science/article/abs/pii/S1036731424002832.

mean that one choice is inherently right and the other wrong, but it does reveal how profoundly grief can shape decision-making in the moment.[30]

That statistic does not haunt me so much as it humbles me. It reminds me that even the most skilled approach cannot override the tidal wave of sorrow crashing over a mother and father in the pediatric ICU. Sometimes the ventilator is the barrier, sometimes it is fear, and sometimes it is simply the limit of human endurance. My role is not to secure an outcome but to walk with them as they discern what they can and cannot carry.

Emily's story has stayed with me, not because of the "no," but because of what it taught me about presence. It taught me that silence can be a gift. Being clinical and clear is an act of mercy. That sitting on the floor with parents as they wrestle with an impossible decision may be the holiest ground I have ever stood on.

In the end, we are not measured by how many "yeses" we receive, but by the mercy we show in every room we enter. Sometimes mercy is helping a family say yes. Sometimes mercy is honoring their no. Either way, the sacredness is the same.

---

[30] J. S. Rodrigue, et al. "Next-of-Kin's Regret and Satisfaction with Organ Donation Decisions: Results from a National Survey." *Critical Care Medicine* 36, no. 1 (2008): 250–256. https://pmc.ncbi.nlm.nih.gov/articles/PMC2588486/.

CHAPTER SEVEN

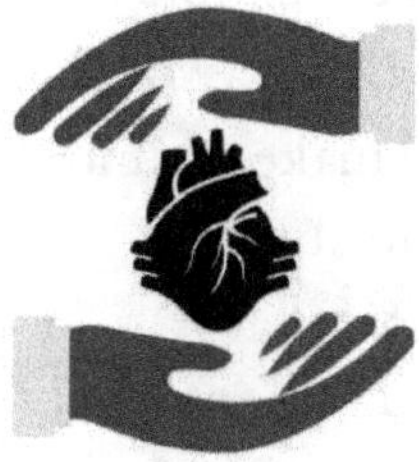

THE ANATOMY OF TIME

"The two most powerful warriors are patience and time."

— Leo Tolstoy

Time.

Everything in the realm of organ donation revolves around it. The timing of the donation conversation—are we entering too soon, or have we waited too long? The timing of the tests that must be completed, the setting of the operating room schedule, the narrow window we are given after withdrawal of life support for a donation after cardiac death to allow for donation to occur.

And above all, there is the question of how much time the family is willing—or able—to wait. Because while we measure time in protocols and procedures, they measure it in heartbreak and endurance. And at some point, time itself becomes the breaking point.

Donor families are the strongest people I have ever encountered. We meet them on what is likely the worst day of their lives—at the moment they have gathered the courage to make an unbearable decision: to turn off the ventilator, or to withdraw life support.

And then, into that fragile moment, I enter with a request that feels impossibly large. *I need you to wait. I need you to give me time—time so that others may have the opportunity to live.*

The most common objection I hear to donation is about time. Families don't usually object to helping others. In fact, most of them want something good to come out of the worst moment of their lives. But once I start explaining the process, time becomes the sticking point.

Time is the biggest barrier to donation. I've heard it over and over: *"We can't wait any longer." "She's already gone, and keeping her on these machines feels cruel."* For parents and spouses, every extra hour at the bedside feels unbearable. They're already running on fumes—physically drained, emotionally gutted, spiritually exhausted.

But on the other side, donation needs time. We need time to run tests, to evaluate each organ, to search for the right recipients, to line up an operating room and a recovery team. Every step matters because this is about dignity—for the donor, for the family, and for the lives that might be saved.

So that's where I stand most days: right in the middle of that tension. A family desperate for release on one side, and a waiting recipient on the other whose only hope is that we can buy just a little more time.

I see this being the case more often than not. In fact, as I was writing this chapter, I had a case where—while the family was supportive of donation—timing became the issue. And in this situation, it wasn't the time on the ventilator or the process itself that created the barrier, but rather the timing of the donation conversation.

This family had agonized over the decision to withdraw life support. They wrestled with it, carried the weight of it, and when they finally made the decision, the emotional energy it required was immense. It was only after they had settled on withdrawal that I was able to go in and begin the donation conversation.

In the hours and days that followed, the patient's son, Derrick, opened up to me about his feelings around the timing. He wasn't opposed to donation. In fact, he and his family were supportive of the idea, but what weighed on him was the sequence—the way one impossible decision was immediately followed by another.

In other instances, the barrier isn't when the conversation happens, but how long the process itself takes. There are circumstances where we can move quickly and get to the operating room for an organ recovery. It's not ideal, but we can make it work.

The truth is, the more time we have, the better the outcomes. More time means more testing, more matches, more opportunities to place every viable organ. And ultimately, more time often means more lives saved.

But again, this is where donation lives—in that constant tension. Families are counting the hours in grief, desperate for release, while we are counting the hours in logistics, desperate for the chance to save as many lives as possible.

One of the unfortunate realities we encounter is when a family reaches their breaking point and asks us to stop the process. It isn't because they don't want to donate. More often than not, their hearts are still in it. But they have simply reached the limit of what they can carry.

Physically, emotionally, and mentally, they can't go any further. The waiting, the machines, the endless hours have become too much, and at some point, donation feels less like a possibility for healing and more like the very thing keeping them from beginning their grieving.

So they say, "We can't do this anymore. We just need to let go."

And in that moment—after every possibility has been explored, every option weighed, and every ounce of strength poured out—I have to honor their limit. Even when I know that lives may not be saved as a result.

This is never an easy call to make. But part of this work is recognizing that mercy sometimes means pressing forward with donation, and other times, it means advocating on behalf of the family in asking that everything be shut down. Either way, my role is the same: to stand with them in the tension and to honor their decision.

In the hundreds of donors I have walked with, only five families have ever asked us to stop. And I remember each one of them as if it happened yesterday. Each time, I grew and learned more about how to set expectations around timing and how to prepare families for the hero's journey that is donation.

But out of those five, one stands apart. It remains one of the most emotionally challenging cases I've ever carried: difficult because of the donor himself, and difficult because of the family's journey through three long days of uncertainty. Unsure how he ended up dead. Unsure who was with him when the events surrounding his death unfolded.. Unsure how they would ever move forward in life without him.

Rodney was in his early twenties—a young gay man whose conservative Christian family was still learning what it meant to be the parents of a gay child. When I first met Gina and Bill, Rodney's parents, it was clear that they were proud of their son and loved him deeply.

They told me about Rodney's coming out, and about how afraid he had been to tell them. He worried that his parents wouldn't accept him, that love might stop at the edge of truth. But when he finally told them, they made sure he knew that he was loved, fully and without condition.

Gina, a pediatric nurse practitioner at the local children's hospital shared with me how shaken she and Bill had been to learn that Rodney ever doubted their acceptance. "We realized then," she told me, "that we needed to do better at showing love and communicating it out loud."

I got the call in the middle of a severe thunderstorm. The hospital was about an hour from my house, and I was told the patient's family was already at the bedside, preparing to withdraw care. So I grabbed my keys, got in the car, and started the drive.

Knowing time was critical, I called the unit to speak with the nurse. I gave her my ETA and asked if she thought the family would be willing to wait. She told me they had been informed that someone was coming to talk with them about next steps. Given the storm, and the fact that it might take me a while to get there, the family had agreed to wait.

By the time I pulled into the hospital, the storm had only gotten worse. I may have driven through a tornado on the way in—whatever it was, itwas bad enough that I felt relieved just to be safe inside the building.

I went straight up to the unit, had a brief huddle with the care team, and then walked into the room to meet the family. I offered to move the conversation into a private conference room, but they declined. They wanted to stay close to Rodney.

"Again, my name is Brent," I said, "and I'm part of the end-of-life care team. I'm here to talk with you about next steps."

There are so many things that could be said in that moment. But I've learned that every word matters. My goal is always the same: to help the family understand the weight of what is to come. Every phrase I choose, every response I give, carries that intentionality.

"Do you mind if I sit with you?" I asked.

"Please," Gina said softly. "My husband will be right back."

"We can wait for him before we begin," I offered. "But while we wait, would you mind telling me what happened to Rodney?"

Gina let out a heavy sigh, fighting back tears as she tried to hold herself steady. "You'll have to forgive me. I'm not even sure where to begin. It's all just so much." She paused, gathering herself. "We love our son. He's gay," she said, her voice firm, almost proud. "We're okay with that. He didn't think we would be, and it devastated Bill—my husband—that Rodney thought we wouldn't still love him. But we did. And we do. I'm just... I'm devastated beyond words that someone would do this to him."

She hesitated, then added, "We think he met someone on one of those dating apps."

At this point, before continuing with the details, I need to pause the story and offer a disclaimer.

Note to Readers: The following section contains references to sexual assault and homophobic language. These details are difficult, but they are part of the truth of Rodney's story. I share them with care, knowing that they may be painful to read.

Bill walked into the room, and I stood to greet him. "Hi Bill, my name is Brent. I was just learning from your wife about what happened to Rodney."

He nodded quietly and took a seat as Gina continued.

"Housekeeping found him," she said, her voice breaking. "He was unconscious and didn't have any clothes on. We got a call from the ER saying he had been brought in. They were waiting on the lab work to see if there were any drugs in his system. When we arrived at the hospital, we were met by the ER doctor—and then detectives who wanted to speak with us. We were confused at first, but they led us into a private room and told us what had happened. They said housekeeping found him naked, with the f-slur written across his forehead. There were signs of sexual and physical assault, and they were getting a warrant for the surveillance footage at the hotel."

My heart sank. "I am so sorry," I said gently. "I can't even begin to imagine what you're going through."

"Thank you," Bill replied, his voice heavy. "I just can't believe he's gone."

Gina stepped in, her voice trembling. "Rodney always was the life of the party. He liked to have fun and always made sure everyone around him felt welcome. I'm so sorry that whoever did this couldn't see his spark the way everyone else did."

She wiped her eyes but pressed on. "We're believers. We know that God loves all of us and wants what's best for His children. But why does stuff like this happen?"

That's the question I ask myself all the time, I thought silently. It's the tension you live with as a trauma chaplain every day you walk into a hospital room. I wish I had an answer. But after multiple degrees in theology, and over two decades in ministry, I still don't.

"I wish I could tell you something that would take away the pain," I said gently. "But what I hold onto—the comfort I find—is knowing that we will all be reunited again. That's the hope we have in the resurrection."

Bill looked at me closely. "Are you a pastor?"

"I'm a chaplain," I replied.

"I could tell there was something special about you," Gina said softly. Then she straightened a little, her voice steadier. "And what were those things you needed to talk to us about?"

"Typically, before I start, I like to make sure families have a good understanding of what the doctors have shared," I said gently. "But I was told on the way in that you're a nurse practitioner—is that right?" I asked, looking at Gina.

She gave a small nod. "Yeah. I work at Children's Hospital in the ICU. You're with the organ procurement organization, right? I thought you looked familiar." A faint recognition flickered across her face. "I was wondering when you all were going to come talk with us."

"Bill," I said, turning toward him, "I want to make sure you don't have any questions before we move forward with discussing Rodney's opportunity to save lives through donation."

He shook his head gently. "I think I have a good understanding from what was explained to me earlier. It's helpful being married to an NP—she's been my rock through all of this."

"Have you had the chance to talk together about how you'd want to proceed?" I asked.

"Is he registered?" Gina asked quickly. "We couldn't find his driver's license to check, because they have all of his belongings in evidence."

"One of the first things I did when I arrived," I explained, "was pull his BMV record. He's not registered."

Gina's shoulders slumped. "I was hoping he was—so we wouldn't have to make that decision."

"I understand," I said gently. "There are any number of reasons why someone might not be registered. The most common is simply that no one asked at the time he got his license."

I paused, then leaned in. "Bill and Gina, you knew Rodney best. If I were able to ask him right now—if he knew he had the chance to save up to eight lives through organ donation and enhance countless others through tissue donation—what would he say?"

Bill didn't hesitate. "He would say yes."

I turned to Gina. She nodded, though her face tightened. "He definitely would say yes. I'm just… concerned, though."

"What are your concerns?" I asked.

She took a deep breath. "Rodney liked to hook up a lot, and I'm not sure he was always safe when he did. What if he has an STI?"[31]

"That's a good question," I said. "We actually do a full medical screening on every donor to make sure there's nothing that could be passed on to a recipient. Even if something does come back, like hepatitis, a recipient can choose whether or not to move forward. If they accept, there are antivirals and treatments that they can be placed on.

And even patients who are HIV positive, or living with AIDS, can still be donors. They donate to recipients who are also HIV positive, so those lives can still be saved."

Gina looked up, surprised. "Even people with HIV?"

"Even people with HIV," I said gently. "There's actually a federal law called the HOPE Act. It was passed to allow people living with HIV and AIDS to both donate and receive transplants safely. It means that what once would have been ruled out as impossible is now giving people a second chance at life."

Early on in my career as a donation advocate, I learned about the HOPE Act. For decades, HIV was an automatic exclusion in donation and transplantation. If a potential donor tested positive, the case would immediately be shut down, even if the donor was otherwise perfectly healthy. But this was one of those medical lines in the sand that no one thought would ever be crossed. But in 2013, Congress passed the HIV Organ Policy Equity (HOPE) Act, which allowed organ donation between

---

31 *STI stands for sexually transmitted infection, an infection that is passed from one person to another through sexual contact. Common examples include HIV, chlamydia, gonorrhea, and syphilis.*

people living with HIV. Suddenly, people who had once been excluded—people who had been told their lives couldn't give life—were given the chance to both donate and receive.

The impact has been incredible. Since the first HOPE Act transplant in 2016, countless lives have been saved, and it's estimated that allowing HIV-to-HIV transplantation could add hundreds of transplants each year. To me, the HOPE Act is more than just a piece of legislation. It's a reminder that medicine evolves, that what was once impossible or unthinkable can become a new frontier of healing. And it's also a reminder of dignity—that every person, no matter their diagnosis, deserves the chance to give life and to receive it.

Gina looked at Bill. "I think we should do it."

"I agree," he said.

"Thank you both so much," I replied. "There's just some paperwork we need to complete, and then we can get started."

Together we went through the forms—the authorization for donation and the Universal Donor Risk Assessment Interview, or UDRAI. Once everything was signed, we wrapped up the paperwork and parted ways.

As I left the hospital, I realized I needed to stop for gas. There was a station just across the street. As I stepped out of my car, I glanced back toward the hospital and saw a rainbow arching overhead. I snapped a picture and sent it to Gina and Bill.

Within minutes, Gina responded: *"I think it's Rodney letting us know that we did the right thing."*

The next day I went back to the hospital to check in on both the case progression and on Bill and Gina. We sat together for a while, just visiting, and I let them know that things were moving forward. They hadn't received any updates from the detectives, so the unanswered questions still weighed heavily on them.

I shifted the focus, as I often do, to memory-making. I helped them record Rodney's heartbeat and placed it inside a small bear for them to keep. I also presented them with the Donor Hero Medal—a simple token, but one that carries deep meaning for families who need to know their loved one is remembered with honor. Before I left, I reassured them that I would check in as soon as we had an operating room time scheduled.

The following day I learned that we had entered the allocation phase of the donation process—when the clinical team begins working to find recipients. I stayed on site, waiting for Gina and Bill to arrive so I could update them in person. When they walked in, I could see the strain written on their faces. They still hadn't heard anything from the detectives, and the waiting was starting to wear them down.

I explained where we were in the process and told them the operating room would likely be scheduled for the next day. I promised that by the end of the day I should have the exact time.

That evening the call came in: the OR was set for the following day at 1800—6:00 p.m. I went into the room and shared the update with Gina and Bill. They nodded, grateful for clarity at last.

"Thank you," Gina said softly. "I'm tired, and I'm just ready to start the next chapter of all of this."

"I can imagine," I said quietly. "I appreciate you both so much—and your willingness to walk this journey with us. I'll be here tomorrow to support you. If there's anything you need overnight, please don't hesitate to let me know."

By day three, Gina and Bill looked completely exhausted. They were ready for it to be over. And yet, in their exhaustion, you could see the pride shining through. They were proud of their son—proud of who he was, proud of the life he had lived, and proud of the gift he was about to give.

I checked in with my clinical team. "Still on for 1800?"

Then came the words you never want to hear as a donation advocate: *"We've been bumped back to 1900."*

"Okay," I thought. "An hour isn't too bad. I can talk to Bill and Gina—they'll understand."

I spoke with them, and they took it in stride. I let my clinical team know we were fine.

But then 1800 rolled around, and my coordinator's phone buzzed. *"OR is delayed. A trauma just came in."*

This happens often at a Level 1 trauma center, and we prepare families for it as best we can. Still, I had to walk back to Bill and Gina and tell them that we'd been delayed again—that the team would get us into the OR as soon as possible.

By 2000, I could feel myself getting antsy and frustrated. My family had already endured so much, and now the recovery had been bumped twice.

I turned to my clinical coordinator and said, "I need a set time. We cannot keep going back to this family with shifting updates. Call whoever you need to call, escalate it as high as it has to go—but we need something in stone." She agreed and started making calls, pushing it up to our leadership.

The answer came back from the hospital: they wouldn't commit. Too many procedures had already been bumped. They couldn't give us a firm time—or even confirm if the recovery would happen at all that day.

Then came the hardest part. I was asked to go back to Bill and Gina yet again and ask them for more time.

I walked into the room slowly. "Bill, Gina," I began, "I'm so sorry. We're having trouble getting a set OR time for Rodney's recovery. I've escalated it to my leadership, and they've escalated it to the hospital leadership, but right now we still don't have a guarantee."

Bill shook his head. His voice was heavy. "Brent, we can't do this anymore. I'm sorry, but we just can't."

Gina reached over and touched his arm. "They have until midnight," she said firmly. "Bill, we'll give them until midnight. But if it's not done before then, we're canceling it."

I nodded. "That is more than fair."

I brought their decision back to my leadership and my clinical team. Conversations continued with the hospital, but the response was the same: they could not guarantee us a time.

Those last hours seemed to fly by, and soon we were approaching 2300. The OR control desk still couldn't give us a time. The next sixty minutes felt like the most agonizing of all—sitting with the family, minute by minute, waiting for the phone to ring.

The call never came. At 23:59, Gina looked at me with tears in her eyes and said, "I'm sorry, Brent, but we have to stop now."

I apologized to Gina and Bill, thanking them for their willingness to walk this journey with us, even though donation could not happen. We informed our leadership that the case was shutting down, packed up, and went home. Bill and Gina stayed behind, spending a few quiet hours with Rodney before the machines were finally shut off.

A week later, I was at home getting ready for my daughter's softball game when my phone rang. It was Gina.

"Hi, this is Brent, how may I help you?" I answered.

Her voice broke on the other end. "Hi Brent, this is Gina. I just wanted to call and apologize… for not seeing this through. I think we made a terrible mistake by not allowing Rodney to be a donor. I'm sorry we weren't strong enough to let it happen."

"Gina," I said gently, "it's okay. If anyone should be apologizing, it's me—for not being able to meet your timeline requests. I'm sorry we couldn't make this happen. But I want you to know something: we consider Rodney a donor hero in spirit. The gift was in the yes. The system failed—but you didn't. You had no control over that."

Through her tears, she whispered, "Thank you, Brent. That means a lot to me."

Time. It's the one element I can never control, no matter how hard I try. In every donor case I've ever walked into, time is the constant thread running beneath it all—the urgency of medicine, the exhaustion of families, the ticking of the clock inside a trauma center. Sometimes time feels like a gift, giving families a chance to gather, to make memories, to say goodbye. And other times, time feels like the greatest enemy, stretching families to their breaking point until they can no longer carry the weight of waiting.

I think back to Gina and Bill. For three days, I watched them wait. Wait for detectives. Wait for answers. Wait for their son's belongings to be released from evidence. Wait for an operating room that never seemed to open. I watched them wear the grief on their faces—first as strength, then as patience, and finally as sheer exhaustion. They loved Rodney deeply, and they wanted his story to ripple out into the lives of others. But by the end, time became the very thing that kept them from carrying through. Their willingness was there. Their desire to honor their son was there. But their strength to keep waiting was gone.

This is the tension we live in as donation advocates. On one side, I know the medical reality: the longer we have to test, allocate, and plan, the more lives can be saved. More time means more transplants. More time means fewer wasted gifts. More time means hope extended to the people waiting on the other end of the line. But on the donation side of things, there is the donor family—the ones who are sitting in the ICU chairs for hours upon hours that bleed into days, sleeping in hospital waiting rooms, holding onto the last physical moments they will ever have with someone that they love. For them, this time isn't measured in labs or testing, in matches, or in logistics. It's measured in sighs, in tears, in the painful heartbeat of anticipation. And at some point, the waiting breaks them.

I've seen families give me the gift of time. They've said yes, even when it meant waiting one more night, or putting off the funeral arrangements, or watching their loved one on a ventilator when every instinct told them it was time to let go. And I've also seen families who, after waiting as long as they possibly could, finally said, "We can't do this anymore. We just need to let go." In those moments, it's not a rejection of donation—it's a recognition of human limits. Mercy means honoring that limit, even when I know what could have been saved.

Someone once told me that time was a predator that stalked us all our lives. But I rather believe that time is a companion who goes with us on the journey, and reminds us to cherish every moment… because they'll never come again."

— Captain Jean-Luc Picard, *Star Trek: Generations*

Time is not neutral in this work. The weight of it presses on everyone—the control desk nurses who are trying to keep operating room schedules open, our organ recovery coordinators who are running labs through the night, the donation advocates like me who stand in the tension between logistics and compassion. But most of all, it presses on families. They didn't ask for the clock to start ticking. They didn't sign up for this race against time. They only want their loved one to live. And when that isn't possible, all they want is the chance to grieve.

The truth is, the best-laid plans in donation can be undone by the clock. An OR gets bumped. A trauma comes in. A family breaks under the strain of waiting. And no matter how hard we fight, there are times we lose the chance to turn one yes into life for others. That reality hurts. It stays with you. I can still see the five families who told me to stop after they had said yes. Five families out of hundreds. Five stories etched into my memory. Each one taught me something about time, about patience, about setting expectations, and about the sacred responsibility of walking with families as far as they are able to go.

Rodney's case still lingers with me more than most. Maybe it's because of who he was—a young man whose parents loved him fiercely, who had to wrestle with being himself in a world that often wasn't kind. Maybe it's because of the storm that night, the rainbow over the hospital, the way Gina told me she thought it was Rodney's way of letting them know they made the right choice. Or maybe it's because of the way time stole from them the chance to follow through on their yes. Whatever it was, I'll never forget the mixture of exhaustion, pride, and love I saw in his parents' eyes as they finally said, "We're ready to start the next chapter."

And then there was Gina's call a week later. Through tears, she apologized for not letting Rodney be a donor, as if she had failed him. I told her what I truly believe: that Rodney is a donor hero in spirit. His parents said *yes*. Their hearts said *yes*. Their faith said *yes*. The fact that the system and the clock didn't cooperate doesn't take away from the gift they were willing to give. That willingness itself is a kind of donation. It's a gift to me, to the team, to every recipient who lives with hope that families like theirs exist.

Time will always be part of the story. Families measure it one way, hospitals another, and advocates like me walk in between the two. I've had to learn to live with that tension, to prepare families for it, and to show mercy when it becomes too much. I've also had to learn to forgive myself when time steals something from us that no amount of advocacy could secure.

As I think back over the hundreds of families I've met, I can honestly say that time has been both the greatest enemy and the greatest teacher. It has taught me patience. It has taught me humility. It has taught me to sit longer in silence, to prepare families better for what's ahead, and to accept that sometimes the most merciful thing is to let go.

In the end, time forces me to face my own limits. I can't control the OR. I can't control the clock. I can't control when a family breaks. What I can control is the way I show up in those moments—the way I choose my words, the way I sit in silence, the way I hold both grief and hope in the same breath.

Time will always create tension in this work. But tension doesn't mean failure. Tension means humanity. It means that in the middle of loss and logistics, love still matters more. Families still matter more. Presence still matters more. And maybe that's the lesson of time—that it isn't ours to master, but to honor.

As I close this chapter, I don't offer a neat answer. Time will always frustrate, it will always push, and it will always test. But time also has a way of reminding us all of why this work matters. It's because, in those hours that feel unbearable, in those nights that stretch far too long, it is in those moments when a family says yes or no, that time is what holds the sacred space between life and death. And in that space, we are called to show up—with mercy, with presence, and with the courage to honor every single moment for what it is.

CHAPTER EIGHT

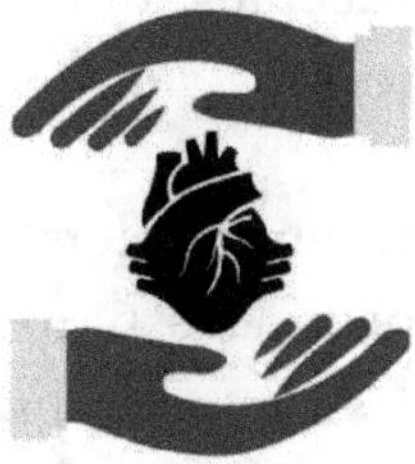

THE ANATOMY OF LEGACY

"What you leave behind is not what is engraved in stone monuments, but what is woven into the lives of others."

— Pericles

Legacy is not an abstract idea in the world of donation. It is measured in heartbeats, in breaths, in meals shared around a family table. Every gift given becomes another life carried forward, another story that continues.

I often think of it this way: for every heart transplanted, there are roughly 37 million additional heartbeats each year.[32] Every lung transplanted equals nearly 8 million breaths annually.[33] Every kidney transplanted means thousands of gallons of blood filtered, toxins cleared, and years added to someone's life. A liver transplant processes hundreds of meals, turning food into energy and keeping someone strong enough to embrace their children or walk into work.

This is what legacy looks like when you translate it into the language of the body. It isn't just numbers—it's birthdays celebrated, graduations attended, grandchildren held, songs sung, prayers whispered, and laughter that never would have been heard without the gift of donation.

I remember a donor's mother once telling me, *"I count my son's legacy in the birthdays that are still happening because of him."* That has stayed with me. Her son's heart now beats inside another chest. His lungs now breathe for someone else. His kidneys filter blood for another family's father, another family's brother. To her, the legacy wasn't about how her son died—it was about how he continued to live.

That is the anatomy of legacy: a rhythm of continuation, measured not only in medical terms, but in the very ordinary and sacred moments that ripple outward from one "yes."

That's what donation really is at its core. A ripple that moves forward through time, brushing up against people you'll never meet. It's one family saying goodbye while another family gets to say hello again.

---

32 *Based on an average human resting heart rate of ~70 beats per minute, multiplied across one year.*

33 *Based on an average adult respiratory rate of ~15 breaths per minute, multiplied across one year.*

Every heartbeat, every breath, every step a recipient takes belongs to that ripple. And the thing is, the legacy doesn't stop in the operating room. It spills out into kitchens and classrooms, into hospital waiting rooms and church pews. A dad makes it to his daughter's graduation. A grandma gets to rock her grandbaby. A mom lives long enough to see her son walk down the aisle.

Most of the time, we'll never see those ripples with our own eyes. But they're there. And for the families who say yes in the middle of the worst day of their lives, that legacy is what ties loss to life, grief to hope, and memory to meaning.

The donor hero who, to me, showed the truest meaning of legacy was Michael. Michael was a young father of five and a high school soccer coach. He was the kind of coach who wasn't content just to whistle from the sidelines—you'd find him out on the pitch in one-on-one drills with his players, pushing them to be better while laughing right along with them.

He was the picture of health and fitness, the kind of man people assumed would live forever. But more than that, he was loved. Loved by his community, loved by his players, and loved by his family. At the high school, he was almost larger than life—not only because of the championships and undefeated seasons, but because he was carrying on a legacy. He was the second generation in his family to coach that same soccer team, building on what his father had started.

I often tell families that for donation to happen, all the stars in the universe have to line up. The truth is, it's rare. Only about three percent of people who die ever meet the medical criteria to be eligible donors. And even then, there are so many pieces that have to fall into place—the timing, the hospital, the testing, the match.

On top of that, most families have never had a real conversation about donation with their loved one. Death is still a taboo topic in this country, something we avoid until it's right in front of us. Which means when that moment comes, families are often left guessing what their loved one would have wanted.

That's what makes every single donor hero remarkable. It isn't just that they gave organs or tissue—it's that their life intersected with that one-percent window where donation was even possible. Think about it: the same universe that seemed so cruel in taking them too soon, also bent just enough to allow their story to go on through others.

And that's why I always say donation isn't just about science or logistics. It's about alignment. It's about grace. It's about the way tragedy and hope can exist in the same breath. For the families who say yes, their lovedone's legacy becomes proof that even in death, life has the final word.

I was called to the hospital for a donation conversation and, on the way in, I skimmed through the notes. The patient was just a few years younger than me. His wife was bedside. He had been transferred from another hospital.

When I arrived, I learned his name was Michael. That morning, as he was at work, a brain aneurysm ruptured. His wife, Megan, was still in shock as she told me the story. The day had started like any other. She was rushing to get the kids ready for school and daycare. Mikey—as she affectionately called him—was in the bathroom shaving, showering, putting on his work clothes. Before leaving, they kissed goodbye. He headed out the door, and she followed soon after with the children.

There was no warning. No sign that their lives were about to change forever. Megan said she got the call mid-morning—Michael had collapsed. At first, she thought maybe he had passed out or slipped at work. She raced to the hospital hoping for the best, only to be told that he was being transferred to a larger facility that could better manage his care. By the time she made it there, the words *aneurysm* and *rupture* had already entered her vocabulary. Words she never wanted to know. Words that now defined her reality.

She sat at his bedside, staring at the machines that kept him alive. "It doesn't feel real," she whispered to me. "This morning he kissed me goodbye." She shook her head as if replaying it over and over again in her mind, trying to find the point where it all went wrong. "We were supposed to go to the kids' game tonight. He promised he'd bring the snacks. How is this even possible?"

The truth is, I don't have answers. Families don't need me to. What they need is for me to sit there with them, in the middle of the storm, and not run away when it gets heavy.

That's how it was with Megan. There wasn't anything I could say that was going to make losing Michael easier, so I didn't try. I just sat close, listened, and let her talk when she could. Sometimes that's the whole job—just being there and not flinching.

At some point, I had to bring up donation. That's why I was there. But it's never about pushing or persuading. It's about listening, giving space, and then saying, *"This is something Michael can do if you want. It's here if you're ready."*

Legacy isn't just about what gets transplanted. It's about the stories families tell, the love they keep saying out loud, and the hope that somehow keeps showing up even in the middle of the worst moments.

So I made the transition. "Megan," I said, "I'm here to talk with you about some important decisions around Michael's legacy."

She nodded, eyes red and tired, but she leaned in, ready to hear me out.

I continued, "Michael has the opportunity to save lives through organ donation. His heart, his lungs, his kidneys, his liver—these gifts could go on to give other families more time with the people they love. It means that even in the middle of this tragedy, his story doesn't stop here. It carries forward."

Megan took a long breath, and then she said something that stopped me. "You know, just this past weekend, we were watching a medical drama that talked about organ donation, and Michael looked at me and said, *'Babe, if something ever happens to me, I'd want to be a donor.'* That's the only reason I'm even considering this right now."

Her voice broke as she spoke, but there was strength in it too. I leaned in a little closer. "Megan, thank you for sharing that with me. That's powerful. He told you what he wanted. You don't have to wonder. You're carrying out his decision, not making it for him."

She nodded slowly, the weight of it still heavy, but something in her posture softened. "So even though he's gone… he can still help?"

"Yes," I said softly. "He can still help. He can still give. He can still make sure other families don't have to go through this same pain."

Can I have some time to think about this and call his parents?" Megan asked, her voice trembling.

"You absolutely can," I said. "Take all the time you need. If you want me to join the call and answer their questions, I'm happy to do that. But I'll be right out at the nurses' station whenever you're ready to talk again."

She nodded that she understood, her hands squeezing the edge of the blanket like it was the only thing left in the room. There was a long silence. The beeps of the machines playing in the background, the steady rhythm of ventilator breaths filling in the silence between us. I've sat in those moments enough times to know not to rush them. Families need them. I needed them too.

"His parents are going to want to know everything," Megan finally said, half to herself. "They're going to ask me why I'm even considering this."

I leaned in a little. "You can tell them what you told me—that Michael told you himself, just a few days ago, that this was what he wanted. That makes all the difference. You're not making this decision for him. You're honoring what he already decided."

Her eyes welled up again. "It's just so fast. We kissed goodbye yesterday morning, and now..." She stopped mid-sentence, covering her face with both hands.

"I know," I said quietly. "It's not fair. None of this is. It's not supposed to happen like this. And I wish I had words that could make it lighter, but I don't. What I can tell you is that you're not alone in this. You've got a team here walking with you."

For a moment, I thought she might collapse under the weight of it all. But she straightened, wiped her tears with the back of her hand, and looked me in the eye. "He'd say yes. I know he would. I just need his parents to hear that too."

"Of course," I said. "They deserve to hear it from you. And if they have doubts or questions, I'll be right there. You don't have to carry that conversation by yourself."

She nodded again, this time with a little more resolve. "Thank you."

As I stood to leave the room, I paused at the door. "Megan, I want you to know something. Whatever you decide, whether you say yes or no, you will have done right by Michael. Because you're sitting here, in the hardest moment of your life, and you're trying to love him well. That's what matters most."

She nodded slowly, and for the first time since I walked in, I saw just the faintest trace of relief cross her face. Not because the decision was any easier, but because she knew she wasn't being forced into it. She knewshe had space.

I stepped out and went back to the nurses' station, giving her the room and the quiet she needed.

I've learned over the years that sometimes the most sacred part of this work isn't the conversation itself, but the pause that follows—the silence where families sit with grief, memory, and the possibility of legacy. It's in that silence that decisions take shape.

So I waited.

After about an hour, Megan came to the nurses' station. Her voice was steady, though her eyes were red. "We all think we would like to move forward with the donation," she said. "What do we have to do?"

I nodded and gently walked her through the process—how we would complete the paperwork, the evaluations, and then the recovery. I tried to make it clear without overwhelming her, step by step, so she could take it in.

As we were talking, I noticed movement at the entrance to the ICU. A group of teenagers had gathered, their faces pale and stunned. Word had spread about what happened to Michael, and his students had started to show up.

The moment Megan saw them, she broke. Tears poured down her face. These were *his kids*—the soccer players that he had coached, mentored, and poured his energy into. Seeing them standing there in the hallway, broken and searching for answers, made the weight of his loss crash over her all over again.

Megan walked over to the students, her own tears still fresh on her face. She didn't try to hide them. She spoke softly, telling them what had happened, her voice breaking as she called him *Coach*.

A heavy silence filled the space, the kind that settles in when the reality finally sinks in. Some of the kids cried openly, others just stared at the floor, their eyes glassy and distant. Grief hung in the air like a weight no one could shake.

One by one, they began to leave—quietly, reluctantly—each carrying the ache of realizing their Coach was really gone. The sound of their footsteps fading down the hall was almost louder than the silence they left behind.

Several days later, we were preparing for the organ recovery. We knew the honor walk would be well attended—Michael was beloved—and both we and the hospital had called in extra staff to help support the people who would come.

But nothing could have prepared me for what we walked into. I have never seen so many people gather for an honor walk. The hallways were lined with faces—students in their soccer uniforms, coaches, teachers, family, friends, neighbors, and people from the community who simply wanted to be there. The crowd stretched so far that I wondered if there would even be enough space in the corridor to hold them all.

It wasn't just a hospital hallway anymore. It felt like a stadium tunnel, filled with the quiet reverence of a community united in love and grief.

Michael went on to save four people through his gift of lungs, liver, kidneys, and heart, and his legacy lives on in each of those individuals. But it doesn't end there.

Every breath they take, every mile they walk, every hug they give to their own families—Michael is part of that now. His five children will grow up knowing their dad's story didn't stop in that hospital room. His players will remember the coach who poured into them and then, in death, poured into strangers he would never meet. His community will carry the memory of that honor walk, when an entire town came together to say goodbye and to bear witness to what love looks like at its deepest level.

That's what legacy is. It's not just four lives saved—it's the hundreds, maybe thousands of lives touched through them. And it's the story that will keep being told, every time someone remembers Michael, not for how he died, but for how he gave.

In addition to the lives Michael saved through donation, Megan has worked to make sure his legacy carries on in their community. She created a foundation in his name—one that pays the fees for student athletes at their school and in neighboring communities.

Michael was never a fan of "pay to play." Every year he would quietly set aside money to cover the cost for kids whose families couldn't afford it, because he believed talent and heart should never be limited by money. Now, thanks to Megan and her tireless work, that same generosity continues. His legacy lives on not only in the recipients who carry his gifts, but in every young athlete who steps onto the field because of the scholarship that bears his name.

When I think about legacy, I think about Michael. His story doesn't end with the aneurysm. It doesn't end with the machines in the ICU. It doesn't even end with the honor walk, though that moment will stay with me for the rest of my life. His story continues every time one of his recipients takes a breath, every time one of his children steps onto that soccer field, every time a kid in his community laces up their cleats because the foundation created in his memory paid their fees.

Legacy is bigger than we think. We often measure it by accomplishments—by trophies, by bank accounts, by titles—but in donation we see legacy for what it really is: a ripple. A heartbeat that doesn't stop when the body does. A breath that carries forward. A gift that multiplies long after the giver is gone.

When I walk with families, I remind myself that most of them have never thought about legacy in this way. For them, the word usually feels abstract. But when they say yes to donation, they put flesh and bone to it. They take something theoretical and make it visible. And that yes doesn't just live in medical charts or transplant records—it lives in stories, in communities, in the ordinary moments that happen because someone else gave them the chance.

A transplanted organ doesn't just function — it gives time. Time for morning cups of coffee, late-night conversations, school drop-offs, family traditions, and the thousands of ordinary moments that make a life feel whole again.

Michael's legacy lives in those numbers, yes, but more than that, it lives in the people who get to keep telling their stories because of him. That's the gift. That's the miracle of it all.

But legacy is not always easy for families to see right away. In the middle of grief, it's hard to imagine anything beyond the rawness of loss. I've sat with moms and dads who couldn't even form the word "donation" without sobbing. I've stood in rooms where silence spoke louder than words. I've been looked in the eye and told "no." And those refusals are part of the legacy, too. Because even when donation doesn't happen, the love, the struggle, the willingness to even sit with the question—those are seeds planted in the soil of legacy.

What I've learned over the years is that legacy isn't a moment. It's a story that keeps unfolding. It's Megan standing in the hallway with her husband's players, holding their grief as much as her own. It's the foundation she started in his name, making sure no child in her community is sidelined because their parents can't afford the fees.

And legacy shows up in quieter ways, too. In the way a family sets an extra place at the holiday table. In the way a widow keeps her husband's laugh alive in stories to their kids. In the way communities rally around each other in those early weeks of grief. All of it matters. All of it tells us that death does not have the final word.

When I think back on Michael's honor walk, what strikes me most isn't the number of people who showed up—though it was overwhelming—it's the reverence in that hallway. Hundreds of people standing shoulder to shoulder, not saying a word, because they knew what was happening was holy. They may not have named it that, but I will. It was holy. A father, a coach, a friend being carried out not only as a patient, but as a hero. A community gathering to witness love in its most costly form.

That's legacy. Not the kind we write on résumés or etch into gravestones, but the kind that keeps beating and breathing in other people.

And here's what I want families to hear: legacy is not about perfection. Michael wasn't perfect. None of us are. Legacy is about what remains when the dust settles. For Michael, it was his heart for his kids, his passion for his players, his commitment to making sure no one was left out. For other donors I've walked with, it has been different—sometimes complicated, sometimes messy. But the beauty of donation is that it gathers all of that up and turns it into life.

I've learned that legacy is often clearest in hindsight. Families may not see it in the ICU, when everything feels unbearable, but weeks, months, years later, they look back and realize that saying yes gave them something to hold on to. As you have read in the previous chapter, I've had moms call me months after saying no, telling me they wished they could go back. I've had dads send me letters of gratitude because their loved one's decision to donate gave them peace. Legacy, in those moments, becomes a lens through which grief can be carried.

For me, as a donation advocate, legacy is also a mirror. It asks me what kind of mark I'm leaving, not just in my work, but in my life. Am I showing up fully for the people in front of me? Am I living in such a way that if today were my last day in this field, would I leave behind more than a line on my résumé? Donation forces me to ask those questions every time I step into a hospital room.

Legacy is not a choice about whether or not we leave one—we all leave one. The choice is what kind it will be. And in donation, families are given the chance to leave a legacy that speaks louder than death. That's the anatomy of legacy: love written into the fabric of other people's lives.

Michael's five children will grow up with the story of their dad not only as a coach and father, but as a hero who gave life to others. His players will always remember the man who taught them discipline and joy, who played alongside them, who believed in them. His community will keep telling the story of the coach who hated "pay to play" and made sure kids got on the field regardless of their parents' bank accounts. And his recipients—though they may never know the man that gave them life—will carry him with every heartbeat, every breath, every step.

That's legacy. That's the ripple. That's the anatomy of a yes.

When I sit with families like Megan's, I'm reminded that my role is not to manufacture legacy but to point to it, to hold it up, to remind them that their loved one's story still matters. I'm there to listen, to guide, to give space for grief and hope to coexist. And in that space, legacy takes root.

In the end, legacy is less about what we accomplish and more about what we give. It's less about what we hold onto and more about what we release. Donation teaches us this better than anything else. It shows us that the most lasting legacies are not built on what we keep, but on what we let go.

And so I think again of Michael. A coach. A father. A donor. A man whose story did not end in a hospital room but lives on in lungs that breathe, a liver that strengthens, kidneys that filter, and a heart that still beats. A man whose love for his players lives on in scholarships. A man whose yes became the beginning of someone else's tomorrow.

That's the anatomy of legacy.

CHAPTER NINE

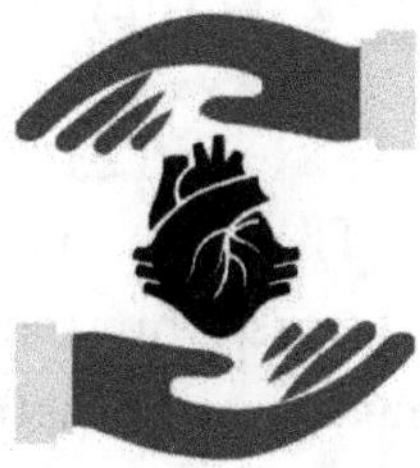

THE ANATOMY OF HOPE

"To plant a seed is to believe in tomorrow."

— Audrey Hepburn

Hope is a word we use a lot in the world of organ donation—especially on the donor side. I spend countless hours each week sitting with families, speaking about the hope that donation offers. The hope that out of their loss, something meaningful might emerge. The hope that a life cut short can still ripple outward in ways that matter.

There is also the hope carried by those waiting for a call that could change everything. The hope that when the phone rings, it will mean that a donor has been found, that they should come to the hospital, that life might be extended. And yet sometimes that hope is met with heartbreak—the organ is found diseased, or the donor does not pass in time, and the possibility evaporates before it ever truly begins.

And then there is my hope—the kind I carry with me into every hospital room and every waiting area. The hope that I am giving the very best of myself to the family sitting across from me, a family who has just lost everything. The hope that my presence matters, even in the shadows of their grief. The hope that my work leaves a mark, that somehow I am making a difference in this field I love so deeply.

I have to be honest: I dreaded writing this chapter. Strange, isn't it? Especially considering its title—*The Anatomy of Hope.* But I dreaded it because writing it meant something more. It meant that this book was nearing its end. Not because this chapter comes last in order, but because it is the final story I've chosen to write. This book has been my companion on long journeys, my outlet when the weight of the work pressed heavily, my escape in the aftermath of hard cases. To close it feels like closing a season of my own life. And, truth be told, I dreaded it because hope is not always easy to write about. Hope is fragile. It is delicate. It is so often born in the cracks of grief and nourished by tears. But that is also what makes it powerful.

Hope is not optimism. Optimism says things will get better. Hope says even if they don't, life still has meaning. Optimism looks for outcomes. Hope looks for presence. Optimism demands answers. Hope lives with mystery.

But I also dreaded this chapter because I hadn't found the right story yet. Hope deserves the right story. Each chapter in this book has been born from the right story, at the right moment, and I owed the same to you, the reader. For this one—maybe the most important of them all—I had to wait until the words came, until the story revealed itself. Only then could I sit down and write these pages.

Because hope, more than anything else, is what keeps me here. It's what keeps families saying yes. It's what keeps patients holding on. And it's what keeps me walking into rooms where grief is louder than words, carrying the fragile belief that even here—even now—hope has a place.

In this work, I have countless conversations about donation, and I meet more people than I could ever possibly keep track of. Every day brings something new. There are the firsts—my first time working with a celebrity donor, my first time navigating a high-profile case splashed across local and national news. Each one of those moments is unique, each one special in its own way, and each one leaves behind a story worth carrying.

And then there is Christopher.

Christopher was 23 years old, a young man with Down syndrome, and as his Aunt Millie told me—more than once—he was the life of the party. He lived in a nursing home because Millie and her husband Patrick weren't able to care for him at home. Millie was in the middle of her own battle with breast cancer. Still, it was obvious to me how deeply they loved him.

I wasn't the one who spoke with Millie and Patrick about the possibility of organ donation. That conversation was handled by a colleague and good friend of mine. I was simply there to support the organ recovery, filling in because my teammate was off. It meant I met Millie, Patrick, and Christopher for the very first time just two hours before the recovery was scheduled to take place.

In those two hours, I saw for myself what everyone else already knew—just how special Christopher really was.

I knocked gently on the door.

"Do you mind if I come in? My name is Brent, and I'm with the organ procurement organization. I'm here to be with you through the withdrawal process."

"Please, come in," Millie said as she rose to greet me.

"There's no need to stand," I told her—but she did anyway. That's how they do things here. Even in the heaviness of grief, respect and kindness are the first things offered.

"I know Isabella already went over things with you," I continued, "but I wanted to review them again, just to be sure you don't have any questions."

I explained the plan: "We'll be moving down to a room just outside the OR. I'll have chairs set up for you there. Withdrawal will take place at 8:00 p.m., and we'll wait up to 120 minutes for Christopher to pass. He will be given all the comfort medications, just as he would if he were here in his room and not going on to be a donor."

Millie's face softened. "Oh, he's happy to be a donor. There was never any question about it when Isabella came and talked to us. Christopher isn't the first in our family to be a donor."

Her words caught me off guard, and my curiosity stirred. There was more to this family's story, and I wanted to understand it.

"He's not?" I asked, surprised.

Millie shook her head gently. "No, he's not. He's actually the third in our family. His momma was a donor when she died, and so was his granddaddy—my daddy."

I paused, letting the weight of her words settle in. *Third generation.* In all my years, I had never encountered something like this. Tragic, yes, but also profoundly beautiful.

"So your family really supports organ donation then," I said softly.

Millie nodded. "My mother's life was saved because of a donor. From that day on, we made a commitment: if the time ever came, we were all going to donate."

"That's truly amazing," I replied. "I really mean it. I've never seen a family with multiple generations of donors before. I can't thank you enough for your willingness and your legacy."

Millie smiled, her eyes bright with memory. "I remember it like it was yesterday. We got the call to come to the hospital—there was a heart for my mother. I was just a teenager, sitting in that waiting room, and let me tell you… you'll never guess who else was in the hospital at the very same time." She leaned in a little, lowering her voice as though to share a secret. She went on to name a well-known country singer who, for privacy's sake, I cannot share here.

"Really?" I said, raising my eyebrows.

"Really. And you'll never guess who showed up to visit them in the hospital that night." She listed off several other prominent country artists, the names tumbling out with the same wonder she had carried as a teenager.

"We tried to catch a glimpse," she laughed, "but we kept our distance. We wanted to give them their privacy, of course."

"That is something else," I responded, shaking my head. "Pretty neat story."

Something seemed to click in Millie's mind.

"Brent," she asked gently, "you said we have 120 minutes to allow Christopher to pass for donation. What happens if… he doesn't?"

I took a breath. This is one of the most challenging aspects of donation to explain. "That's the unfortunate side of this process. If a patient isn't declared brain dead, then they can only be considered a donor after cardiac death. That means once the ventilator is removed, we have a limited amount of time—120 minutes—for the patient to pass. If death doesn't occur in that timeframe, the organs are no longer viable for transplant."

Millie nodded slowly, seemingly taking it in. "Oh, that has to be a terrible feeling for the person waiting on the other side, expecting the organ." She paused, then her eyes grew distant as the memory of her mother's transplant surfaced. "I remember when we were waiting for my mother's transplant. We saw a man coming down the hallway with a red cooler labeled *Organ.* We were so excited, convinced it was her heart. But it wasn't. Her heart didn't arrive until an hour later. I can't imagine what it would feel like if that heart had never come at all."

Her words landed heavy. She understood in a way most families didn't—the fragile tension between hope and heartbreak, between the promise of life and the limits of time.

"Millie, unfortunately, that does happen sometimes," I said gently. "Sometimes a patient doesn't pass in time, or we discover an organ is too diseased to be transplanted. But I've heard from friends who've been on the waitlist that even those false starts matter. Every 'almost' is still a yes from a family. And for someone waiting, knowing that families are willing—it gives them the strength to keep fighting for another day."

"I can't imagine your job is easy," Millie said softly.

I nodded. "It's not," I admitted. "But I find my hope—and my drive to keep going—by working with families like yours. Families who set aside their own needs in the midst of grief to think of others. It's an honor to walk with those families and be even a small part of their story."

This work takes a toll. It asks more of a person than most will ever see. I've watched colleagues burn out, break down, and step away because the weight of grief and responsibility became too much. And I'd be lying if I said I haven't felt that pull myself. Missing my own family's big moments so I can sit with another family in their worst moment—it hurts.

But deep down, I know I'm exactly where I'm meant to be. This is more than a job. It's my vocation. My place.

Several moments later, my clinical teammate came in and told us it was time to begin preparing Christopher for his journey to the OR. Together, we readied him, and then I carefully draped the Donate Life flag over his body for the honor walk.

We began the solemn procession down the hallway, a hush falling as we approached the double doors that led to the prep area of the OR. When we entered the room, Millie turned to me and asked, "Brent, will you lead us in prayer?"

So I did. I prayed the best I could—trying to weave words that would be meaningful for them in their Southern Baptist faith, even as I prayed out of my own Anglican tradition. As I closed with "Amen," I looked up and saw the nurses and clinical staff in tears. They thanked me for the prayer, as did Millie and Patrick.

Then the ventilator was removed, and silence filled the room. In that silence, my own prayer continued—that Christopher would pass peacefully and in time to fulfill the gift his family had said yes to. And he did.

Christopher went on to save multiple lives, continuing not only his family's legacy but also leaving his own indelible mark on the world of donation.

It is donors and families like this that give me hope. Hope is not always easy to hold onto. Turn on the news, and it can feel like hopelessness is everywhere. Current events—especially those critical of donation—can weigh heavily, and sometimes it feels as though the world is against you and the sacred work you are trying to do. That weight finds its way into the conversations we have with families, when they mention the latest article or headline that questions the very thing we are inviting them into.

And yet, that is exactly why our work as donation advocates matters. It is why books like this matter. We have to pull back the veil and let the world see what really happens inside ICU rooms and hospital waiting rooms. We must invite others to witness the sacred conversations, the impossible decisions, and the profound moments of grace that occur every single day.

Because in the end, it is stories like Christopher's—and families like his—that keep hope alive.

Hope. It is such a simple word, only four letters, and yet it carries the weight of the world. In organ donation, it is a word we use constantly. We speak of the hope families find in creating meaning from unimaginable loss. We speak of the hope that those on the waiting list cling to as they count down days and hours, watching their own time slip away while praying that someone else's yes will arrive in time. And I speak of the hope I carry, the hope that I am enough for the families I serve, the patients I never meet, and this vocation that calls me again and again to show up.

Throughout these pages, I have tried to let you into a world most people never see. A world of ICU rooms and waiting areas, of whispered prayers and impossible decisions, of goodbyes spoken in the language of ventilators and monitors. I have tried to bring you to the bedsides and hallways where this sacred work takes place, not to sensationalize it, but to humanize it. Because that is what donation really is—not a process, not a policy, not a transaction. It is human. It is relational. It is sacred ground.

That is what I have learned from donor families in Appalachia and beyond. Families who say yes, not because the outcome is guaranteed, but because it is right. Families who find hope, not in what can be measured or promised, but in what can be given. Families like Christopher's, whose story will forever remain with me.

Christopher was not the first in his family to be a donor. He was the third. His mother before him, his grandfather before her, and now him—continuing a legacy written in yeses. A family shaped by both receiving and giving, by living and losing, by the threads of donation woven into their history. When Millie told me that story, I realized something profound: hope is not just individual, it is generational. It is something passed down like an heirloom. It is a seed planted in one season that blossoms in another.

As I prayed with that family, as I walked with them to the OR, as I watched Christopher's life continue through the lives he saved, I was reminded that hope is not abstract. It has a name, a face, a body. Hope is embodied in donors and in the families who speak on their behalf. It is embodied in recipients who wake up with new hearts and lungs. It is embodied in the quiet prayers of nurses and surgeons. And, somehow, it is embodied in the tears of coordinators and chaplains who carry these stories long after the case has closed.

But hope is not just found in the families who say yes. It is also found in the families who say no. Even there, in their choice, there is a kind of hope. Hope that their boundaries will be respected. Hope that their grief will be honored. Hope that their voice still matters in a system that can feel overwhelming. Saying no is not the absence of hope—it is another form of it. It is the family's way of saying: this is how we will carry meaning forward.

I think often of the families who could not donate because the organs were too diseased, or because time ran out, or because circumstances made it impossible. From the outside, those stories can look like failure. But I have learned to see them differently. I have heard from people on the waitlist who tell me that even hearing about a failed match, even hearing that a family said yes though it didn't work out, gave them strength to keep going. They knew there were people out there willing to give. They knew that generosity was real. And sometimes that was enough to fight another day. That too, is hope.

This work is not easy. It is not glamorous. It is often exhausting. I have missed moments with my own family because I was halfway across the country sitting with someone else's family. I have thought about quitting more times than I care to admit. And yet, deep down, I know I cannot walk away. This is my vocation. This is the place where my heart breaks and also the place where my heart is most alive. To stand at the intersection of death and life, grief and legacy, despair and hope—this is the calling I cannot escape.

And so, I remind myself, sometimes daily, of the conversations I have had. Of the families who told me, after the storm had passed, that they were glad I was there. Of the hands I have held, the prayers I have whispered, the sacred yeses I have witnessed. These are the reminders that carry me into the next hospital, the next family, the next story.

CHAPTER TEN

THE ANATOMY OF APPALACHIA

"Appalachia is a place where hope survives best in the shadows of despair."

— *Harriette Arnow*

When I began writing these field notes, I knew there would have to be a chapter on Appalachia. It isn't just the backdrop of my story. It's not just the setting where cases unfold, or where donor families say yes and no. Appalachia is itself a character. It breathes, it aches, it sings, it carries grief and resilience in equal measure. To write about donation without naming the mountains and hollers, the rivers and coal towns, the small churches and high school ballfields that have shaped me—it would leave the story unfinished.

Appalachia is more than geography. It is a way of life, a culture of kinship and stubborn hope. It is also a place that is marked by barriers: poverty, limited access to healthcare, low health literacy rates, systemic neglect, and generational trauma. In many of my donation conversations, I have seen these barriers appear time and again. They shape conversations, influence decisions, and frame the struggles that families face at the bedside.

I have learned that you cannot advocate for donation in Appalachia without first learning to love Appalachia. You cannot step into a hospital in a rural community and expect families to trust you if you don't first honor who they are, where they come from, and the weight of what they carry.

This chapter, then, is not just a conclusion to the stories told before. It is a summation of what Appalachia has taught me, what it demands of us as advocates, and what it asks of anyone who dares to listen. It is both a reflection and a call to action—for donation, for dignity, for hope in a region that too many have written off.

When people hear "Appalachia," their minds often jump to stereotypes: poverty, coal miners, opioid addiction, broken-down towns. And yes, those realities are here. But they don't tell the whole story. Appalachia is also bluegrass music echoing through the hills, it's front-porch conversations with neighbors, it's food shared when there isn't much, it's faith communities holding each other up when the systems fail.

Still, the barriers are undeniable. I've shared earlier how literacy plays a role—how nearly two-thirds of adults in Appalachia read at, or below, an eighth-grade level. That matters when families are handed a packet of medical information about brain death or asked to sign paperwork full of legal and clinical terms. It matters when the decision before them is literally life and death, and the words on the page feel foreign.

Healthcare access is another barrier. Many Appalachian counties are classified as medically underserved. Hospitals are miles away, specialists even further. For organ donation, that means potential donors often die in smaller hospitals without the infrastructure to manage donation cases, or families who don't have a long history of interaction with healthcare may mistrust the system entirely. That mistrust gets projected onto us, the advocates, the strangers in the room asking for something precious in the midst of loss.

Then there is poverty. Families are worried about funeral costs, missed shifts at the plant, and bills that won't stop coming just because someone died. Poverty presses in on every decision. Even when a family wants to say yes, the emotional and financial exhaustion can feel overwhelming. I've sat with moms who wanted to say yes but couldn't bear the thought of waiting another 24 hours because they couldn't afford to miss another day of work.

Layered on top of these barriers are the cultural narratives of pride and privacy. Appalachians don't like outsiders telling them what to do. They don't want pity; they want respect. And they want to make decisions on their own terms, not because some suit from the city shows up with charts and stats.

These barriers are real. But they are not walls. They are invitations—to slow down, to learn, to listen differently. Appalachia demands that you show up with humility and stay long enough to earn trust.

What keeps me coming back to Appalachia, what keeps me hopeful, is not just the struggle but the strength. There is a kinship here that you don't find everywhere. Families are not just nuclear units—they are webs of cousins, neighbors, church members, "aunties" who may not be blood but are family all the same. When a patient is dying, you don't just find a spouse and kids in the waiting room. You find dozens of people, sometimes more, all gathered because family means more than bloodlines—it means belonging.

That kinship cuts both ways. It can complicate decision-making—too many voices, too many opinions. But it also means that when a family says yes to donation, it is not just one person's decision. It is a communal act, a witness to shared values. I've seen families hold each other up in the ICU, hands joined in prayer, saying, "If this is what she wanted, we will stand by her."

That kind of solidarity is what makes donation possible in places where the odds are stacked against it.

Kinship also shows up in the way communities remember their donor heroes. In cities, a donor's story might make the news for a day and then fade. In small towns, the story lingers. People talk about it in the diner, at church, at Friday night football games. A donor hero's name becomes part of the fabric of the place. Legacy doesn't just live in recipients—it lives in communities that carry the memory forward.

So what does this mean for us? For advocates, for healthcare professionals, for communities outside Appalachia who may not understand why this region matters?

It means we must stop seeing Appalachia as a place to be pitied and start seeing it as a place to be partnered with. We must invest in education that is culturally competent and literacy sensitive.

We must be able to address the practical barriers—funeral resources, meeting transportation needs, support for families who say yes but can't afford the time it takes.

It means telling the stories—stories like Michael's, like Emily's, like Brian's—so that the rest of the world knows that hope lives here, too. Appalachia may not have the same resources as other regions, but it has resilience, and resilience is fertile soil for hope.

Appalachia is not just marked by what is said—it is marked by what is not said. Silence carries power here. It carries power because I have seen the power of it as it shows up in hospital rooms when a donor's loved one stares at the floor, avoiding eye contact, because speaking would break them open. It shows up in communities where talking about death is taboo, where preparing for it is seen as inviting it in. It shows up in conversations about donation when the words get stuck in the throat, because saying "yes" feels like acknowledging the finality of loss.

I've had to learn to sit with that silence, to not rush it, to not fill it with statistics or polished words. Appalachia teaches you that sometimes presence is enough. Sitting in a waiting room, hands folded, letting the family's grief fill the space—that's holy work. Out of that silence, words eventually come. And often, they come with surprising clarity. "He'dwant this." "She was always giving." "We don't want her death to be the end of her story."

This is the paradox of silence: it can be a barrier, but it can also be the soil from which hope grows. Families who hesitate, who struggle, who fall silent—these are often the same families who, when they finally do speak, offer the most powerful yeses. Because their 'yes' comes not out of pressure, but out of conviction that they can make a difference.

One of the most striking aspects of donation in Appalachia is its generational nature. In larger cities, families are often nuclear and transient. But in Appalachia, you'll meet three, sometimes four generations at a bedside. Grandparents who grew up in the hollers. Parents who worked the mines or the factories. Children who are the first in their families to go to college.

Each generation brings its own lens. A donor's grandparents may not trust "the system" at all. Their parents may be torn between honoring their parents and embracing something new. The children may be the ones who say, "Mom, Dad, I think this is the right thing to do." I've seen the decision for donation shift entirely because a 20-year-old granddaughter had the courage to speak up and say, "Papaw always told me he wanted to help people. This is a way we can do that."

Generational dynamics can, and often do, complicate donation conversations, but they can also enrich them. When a family says yes in Appalachia, it is often not just one person's choice—it is the blending of generations, the weaving of stories, the reconciling of past mistrust with future hope. That makes the yes more sacred.

When I look back on my work in Appalachia, what stays with me are not the statistics, but the stories.

These are the kind of stories that don't leave you. They stay lodged in my chest, like stones I carry with me. And I think that's how it should be. Appalachia doesn't let you forget. It demands that you carry the stories with you, that you tell them, that you let them shape the way you advocate.

As a chaplain, I can't help but view Appalachia through a theological lens. The mountains themselves preach. They rise and fall like hymns. They hold both beauty and brokenness—streams that give life, mines that take it. They remind me that resurrection always comes with scars.

Appalachia has been scarred by poverty, addiction, neglect, and exploitation. But like Christ's wounds, those scars are not the end of the story. They become the place where hope breaks in. Families who have been beaten down by loss still find the strength to say yes. Communities that feel forgotten by the outside world still rally around donor heroes. Out of death, life still emerges.

To me, that's the gospel in its purest form. That's resurrection in Appalachia. And every yes I've witnessed here is a testimony to that truth.

Some might ask: why focus on Appalachia at all? Why dedicate an entire chapter, an entire reflection, to this region when donation is a national and global issue?

The answer is simple: because Appalachia is often ignored. It is easy to spotlight donation in cities with major transplant centers, where numbers are higher and stories more visible. It is harder to pay attention to rural hospitals tucked in the mountains, where donor cases are few and far between. But those families matter just as much. Their yes carries the same weight, their grief the same depth, their hope the same brilliance.

If we neglect Appalachia, we not only fail these families—we fail the recipients whose lives might be saved by their gifts. The waitlist doesn't care about geography. A kidney from a coal town in Kentucky can save a life in Cleveland just as surely as one from New York City. The lungs of a teacher in West Virginia can bring breath to a child in Atlanta. Donation connects us all, across state lines and cultural divides. Appalachia matters because lives everywhere depend on it.

So, what do we do with all of this? What do we do with the stories, the barriers, the kinship, the theology of the mountains?

We act.

We act by investing in education that meets families where they are, at their own pace. Literacy-appropriate materials. Honest conversations. Advocates trained not just in clinical details but in cultural humility.

We act by telling the stories. By lifting donor heroes from Appalachia so that the rest of the country sees their worth. By publishing, by speaking, by advocating at every level—from hospital boardrooms to state legislatures.

And we act by remembering. Remembering that every yes comes at a cost, that every family carries a weight, and that our role is not just to secure donation but to honor dignity.

MY CLOSING THOUGHTS

As I close this book, I find myself back where I started: standing in the tension between grief and hope, death and life, Appalachia and the world beyond. These mountains have shaped me. They have taught me to listen to silence, to respect kinship, to honor scars, to carry stories. They have taught me that legacy is not measured in numbers but in love, and that hope is never wasted, even when it doesn't lead to a yes.

The anatomy of Appalachia is the anatomy of us all: broken yet resilient, scarred yet beautiful, dying yet capable of giving life. To be an advocate here is to believe that every yes, every seed planted, matters. To be an advocate here is to believe that the mountains still sing, that the rivers still run, that hope still rises, even in the hardest of places.

And so my call to you, the reader, is simple: show up. Wherever you are—whether in the mountains or the city, in a hospital or a classroom, in your church or your community—show up. Show up with dignity. Show up with mercy. Show up ready to carry stories that are not your own. Show up ready to plant seeds of hope, even if you will never see them bloom.

As I set down these pages, I am mindful that the work is not finished. The truth is—it never will be. Even now, as you read this, somewhere a family is being asked to consider donation.

Somewhere, a mother, father, son, or daughter is facing the hardest decision of their lives. Somewhere, a patient is answering a phone call that could mean a second chance.

This work continues, unbroken, through every yes and every no, through every moment of grief and every flicker of legacy.

Because hope is the thread that outlives us all. It is what carries across generations, from one story to the next, from one life to another. And in Appalachia—as in life itself—hope is always the last word.

When I began this book, I thought I was writing about donation. About the process, the statistics, the clinical realities that shape whether a family says yes or no. And I was. But somewhere along the way, I realized I was also writing about something much larger.

I was writing about Appalachia. About the people who shaped me, the mountains that raised me, the culture that both wounds and heals. I was writing about grief, about how it bends us but doesn't break us. And I was writing about hope — the stubborn kind, the kind that shows up even in hospital waiting rooms, even in silence, even in the shadow of death.

The truth is, this work has never been about me. It has always been about the families who, in their darkest hour, choose to think of someone else. It has always been about the patients who wait, sometimes for years, for a second chance at life. It has always been about the communities that rally around their donor heroes, keeping their names alive long after the funeral.

This book is not an ending. It is a witness. A field note from one man who has been privileged to stand in these sacred spaces. The work continues — long after I close my laptop, long after these pages are printed. Even now, as you read this, a coordinator is stepping into a family conference room, taking a deep breath before speaking. Even now, a family is holding hands, deciding whether their yes will be the last gift their loved one gives. Even now, a phone is ringing on a nightstand, and a patient's life is about to change forever.

So what do we do with all of this? We carry it. We let these stories shape us. We remind ourselves that the gift of life is not just a medical transaction — it is an act of love, courage, and hope. We resist the urge to look away when it's hard. We tell the truth, even when the truth is complicated. We keep showing up.

Because Appalachia has taught me that legacy is not measured in what you build, but in who you love. The people here — with their resilience, their kinship, their silence and their song — have shown me that hope is not naive optimism. It is survival. It is rebellion. It is faith.

And so, as I close, my prayer is simple:

May we honor the families who say yes, and the families who say no.

May we see Appalachia not as forgotten hills, but as a teacher in its own right.

May we carry forward the names and stories of donor heroes so they are never forgotten.

And may hope — fragile, fierce, unrelenting — always be the last word.

This is the anatomy of a yes.

This is the anatomy of Appalachia.

This is the anatomy of hope.

And this is my amen.

ACKNOWLEDGEMENTS

No book is written alone. These field notes may carry my name on the cover, but every page has been shaped by the voices, the stories, and the sacrifices of others. To them, I owe more gratitude than words can hold.

First and foremost, I want to thank the donor families who allowed me to walk with them in their hardest hours. To every mother, father, sister, brother, son, and daughter who trusted me with their stories—thank you. Your willingness to let me stand with you in grief, and your courage to say yes during unimaginable loss, has marked me forever. This book is, in many ways, yours more than mine.

To my colleagues in the world of organ procurement: you are the unseen hands and voices who make life possible for countless strangers. I have had the privilege of serving alongside coordinators, administrators, and advocates who give more of themselves than anyone outside our world could imagine. Your grit, your compassion, and your relentless commitment to the mission continue to inspire me.

To my friends and mentors who taught me to keep showing up: thank you for reminding me that presence is the first gift we offer, and sometimes the only one. Your example has kept me grounded when the weight of the work threatened to overwhelm me.

To Irene — my friend, colleague, and companion on the long road of CPE. We learned this work side by side, finding our footing in chaplaincy one vulnerable encounter at a time. You have become a trusted confidant, a voice of wisdom, and a steady presence in both the hard days and the holy ones.

To my family—Heather, Caitlyn, Isabella, Noah, Madeline, and Abigail—thank you for the countless moments you gave up, so I could be at the bedside of another family. Thank you for forgiving the missed birthdays, late-night phone calls, and interrupted vacations. Thank you for reminding me that the vocation I carry is not just mine, but ours. I pray that, in these words, you can see the legacy of love and hope you've helped sustain

And finally, to Appalachia—the mountains and hollers, coal towns and river valleys, the people and places that raised me—you are not just the backdrop of this story. You are its heartbeat. You have taught me resilience, kinship, silence, and song. You have taught me that hope is not naive optimism, but the stubborn belief that life can still rise from the hardest ground.

www.ingramcontent.com/pod-product-compliance
Lightning Source LLC
LaVergne TN
LVHW022052200926
848481LV00003B/877